The Killir

How to avoid a premature death in the supermarket

PAUL KAYE

To my Mum who knows far more about food than
she realises.

With a special thanks to Jenny and Zoe who
ensured that this project got finished.

TABLE OF CONTENTS

GLOSSARY OF TERMS & ACRONYMS

ASA	Advertising Standards Authority
Big Food	The large corporate food manufacturers
BMI	Body Mass Index
BOGOF	Buy one, get one free (promotional mechanism)
CEO	Chief Executive Officer
CSD	Carbonated Soft Drink
GM	Genetically modified
HFCS	High fructose corn syrup
HSE	Health Service for England
MNC	Multi-national corporations
NHS	National Health Service
PHE	Public Health England
SAD	Standard American Diet
SO-BAD	Standard Obese British-American Diet
SSB	Sugar sweetened beverages

THE KILLING FIELDS

Foreword

I have a confession to make. I started the planning for this book several years ago and then got busy with other things. The draft outline sat gathering virtual dust on the hard drive of my computer to the point where I had almost forgotten about it. It was destined to remain on my ever-increasing list of unfinished projects when the coronavirus came along. Suddenly I, like nearly everyone else in the country (essential workers excepted), found myself with more time on my hands than I knew what to do with. The original premise of the book – how to shop better in the supermarket - also took on increasing significance for two key reasons. Firstly, we all had to start buying more food in supermarkets because we could no longer go out to eat. Secondly, and more disturbingly, evidence emerged that seriously overweight and obese Covid-19 sufferers were far more likely to be hospitalised and more likely to die than people of healthy weight.

Although research at the time of writing is at still an early stage, one study found that the risk of dying from coronavirus was 37% higher in overweight patients. Unfortunately, the insights in this book will arrive too late to help these people, but who is to say in the future there won't be other pandemics? I am convinced that staying within a healthy weight range is achievable for nearly everyone. You are what you eat. More than half of the British diet is ultra-processed food. Our nation's deteriorating health is no coincidence, but it doesn't have to be that way. Yes, we are all going to die at some point, but your longevity and quality of life along the way can be directly influenced by what you put in your shopping trolley. The insights and information in this book, if you choose to heed them, will lead to better food choices and improved health.

Introduction

"What a culture we live in, we are swimming in an ocean of information, and drowning in ignorance."
Peter Morville

Imagine you are 18 years old and for your birthday you are given a brand-new car. It's a beautiful car, perfect in every way, but it comes with a condition. It's the only car you are ever allowed to own. If you crash it or damage it you will be responsible for the repairs and if it's damaged so badly that it can't be fixed then you have to live with the consequences. This is the situation with your own body. In the first few years somebody else is responsible for fuelling your 'car' but as you grow into adulthood then it's all down to you. The human body requires 5-star fuel to run at its optimum level but too many of us are using 1-star petrol, i.e. processed food. The cliché 'you are what you eat' has never been truer for the citizens of the UK and our diet that is literally making us ill.

The title of this book derives from a conversation I once had with the CEO of Sainsbury's, one of the UK's major supermarket chains. At the time I was trying to get my company's product onto his shelves. He used the expression 'the killing fields' to describe the challenge for brands to survive in the brutally competitive retail environment where rate of sale and profit per foot of shelf space determined whether you retained your listing. I have taken the phrase in a more literal sense to point out the hidden dangers that shoppers face from the vast array of products that confront them when they go food shopping. Increasingly we are making the wrong choices in so far as they are making us fat and unhealthy. Some of these decisions are made consciously, some out of ignorance and a large proportion are directly influenced by the advertising and marketing of the food manufacturers. This book is an attempt to redress the balance; to put the power back where it belongs in the hands of the consumers. By doing this we can start to reverse the seemingly irreversible trend of obesity and improve the quality and longevity of lives for millions.

We are fortunate to have some of the best food retailers on the planet. Tesco is arguably the most successful food retailer in the world. Sainsbury's has overcome some ups and downs to re-establish itself as a real force. Asda, Morrisons and Waitrose all have a significant base of loyal customers. Meanwhile our food manufacturers have also led some significant innovations in the world of food. However, as a nation we are facing an obesity crisis and for the first time in living memory, life expectancy amongst some socio-economic groups is starting to fall. The percentage of adults who are classed as obese has risen from single digits in 1980 to 29% in 2019 (Note 1). Childhood obesity is showing an even more worrying trend.

As a senior executive in some of the world's leading food companies, I defended the industry's role in this crisis. The argument ran as follows:

- There is no such thing as bad food – only bad diets
- People need to accept personal responsibility for what they eat

- We only give people a choice, and what we offer is driven by what they choose to buy
- If they want high sugar and high fat products, then that is what we will give them

As for children, the parents, we argued, were responsible for their child's diet, not the manufacturers.

The food industry continues to spout this line of thinking and I think that they even believe it. This book will expose the flaws in that thinking and give you an insider's perspective on the vested interests that are perpetuating and accelerating the obesity crisis. The role of the government also needs examining. Their efforts at regulating the food industry to date have been half-hearted and largely ineffective. This is hardly surprising given that their approach involves consulting with food industry leaders who have powerful PR machines to lobby against changes that might potentially damage their sales and bottom-line profits. The other thing to bear in mind is that government's number one priority is to win your vote and get re-elected, not to reduce your waistline. There have admittedly been some initiatives and attempts at regulation. Do you remember the traffic lights debate? Or the salt reduction campaign? These were two protracted initiatives that the food industry successfully stalled. I should know, I helped with the delaying tactics! If you are looking for quick, decisive action, then I'm afraid government intervention is sadly not the answer. Expecting the government to act quickly and decisively is like asking a Frenchman to skip lunch.

I believe that information is power. By reading this book you will have access to inside information on what's really in the food you buy. You'll also have a unique insight into how the food companies convince you to buy products that will literally shorten your life by making you obese and increasing your risk of terminal diseases such as cancer. For years I have been on the other side of the fence designing marketing strategies to convince you to buy and consume food that is bad for you. I am now the archetypal poacher turned gamekeeper. I will share with you the real, underhand tricks of the trade that are contributing directly to the obesity crisis.

More importantly I will walk with you around a virtual supermarket to show you what to avoid, what to cut down on and what might not be all it seems. Yes, and this may come as a surprise to some, food marketing is not completely truthful. In fact, as you will see, in some instances it is downright misleading and bordering on the unethical.

I will focus on the Top 100 British brands - the bestsellers that shoppers regularly and frequently put in their trolleys. Big brands tend to operate in big categories and the Top 100 generate nearly £25 billion of sales. My approach is not exhaustive, and I will not necessarily cover all major categories, e.g. I don't talk about fresh produce in detail, nor alcohol or tobacco (I have no fresh insight on the well-covered dangers of drinking and smoking). I firmly believe it is our addiction (and I use this word literally) to processed food that is the big issue. Processed food tends to be dominated by larger companies who use their marketing muscle and commercial leverage to drive unhealthy over-consumption. After reading this book a trip to the supermarket will never be the same again. You will be armed with insider knowledge that will help you make better choices and potentially lead a healthier, longer life. First though, let us look into our current reality and the existential threat that the obesity crisis represents.

Chapter 1: The Crisis. Right here, right now

"Let them eat cake" (Qu'ils mangent de la brioche), Marie Antoinette

There seems to be a lot of bad news around at the moment. The consequences of the Covid-19 crisis have created fear and 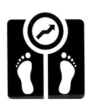 uncertainty, global warming remains a looming threat and Brexit along with the rise of China and other developing economies seems to be relegating Britain to an unprecedented low level in the world standings. Yet, the biggest issue the UK faces as a nation is largely self-inflicted. In the last 25 years obesity rates have more than tripled.

How is obesity measured?

Body Mass Index (BMI) is calculated by dividing your weight (in kg) by the square of your height in metres. A BMI of less than 18.5 means that a person is considered underweight, between 18.5 and 24.9 is considered ideal and 25-29.9 is considered overweight. A BMI of more than 30 means you are obese. If a person has a BMI of over 40 then they would be classed as morbidly obese and well on the way to an early grave.

For some individuals, e.g. elite professional sportsmen and women, BMI is not necessarily a useful or reliable measure. Where such athletes have a combination of extremely low body fat combined with above-average muscle mass, then the BMI can be abnormally high. For most of us, however, BMI is a useful and insightful metric.

If we fast forward to 2050, some forecasters are predicting that the majority of adults and one in four children will be obese. This would represent a disaster for the UK if it came to pass. The health care costs alongside the impact on productivity of an obese workforce would be crippling for our economy, not to mention the social impact of premature deaths and terminal diseases. The current generation of children are potentially the first ever in Britain to have a life expectancy lower than that of their parents.

The latest Health Service for England (HSE) survey published in December 2019 shows that:

- More than half of adults (56%) were at increased, high or very high risk of chronic disease due to their waist circumference and BMI
- 26% of men and 29% of women were obese
- 2% of men and 4% of women were morbidly obese

In Scotland, the figures are even worse with 65% of adults over 16 classed as overweight and 29% (total for men and women) obese. [1]

According to the Department of Health, compared with a healthy weight man, an obese man is:

- five times more likely to develop type 2 diabetes
- three times more likely to develop cancer of the colon

- more than two and a half times more likely to develop high blood pressure – a major risk factor for stroke and heart disease

An obese woman, compared with a healthy weight woman, is:

- almost 13 times more likely to develop type 2 diabetes
- more than four times more likely to develop high blood pressure
- more than three times more likely to have a heart attack

In case the penny hasn't dropped yet, being obese is not going to do much for your longevity let alone your general quality of life while you are still breathing.

We don't need to look any further than the USA for a glimpse of our future if we don't act soon. In 2019, the Center for Disease Control (CDC) found that 36.5% of American adults aged 20 and over, and 17% of American children are obese [2]. This trend has been on-going for decades with no sign of it ending. The number one factor in this epidemic is the food Americans consume: the Standard American Diet (or appropriately enough the SAD) is literally killing people. By way of comparison only 3.6% of Japanese people are classed as obese [3]. Japan coincidentally has one of the highest life expectancies of anywhere in the world. The UK is the most obese nation in Europe, but our near neighbours are also seeing the same trends with France, Germany and Italy tracking at over 20% [4].

There is an old saying that if America sneezes then the UK catches a cold. We have caught the cold. Our dietary habits are following those of the US. This is not surprising given that many of the global food companies are US owned (see Chapter 1) and have transferred their 'best practice' marketing to the UK. There are not surprisingly, however, elements of the British diet that are peculiar to us. Our love of crisps, chocolate bars and sickly sweet baked beans is unrivalled globally and we cannot resist a bit of cheddar cheese whilst the Americans have been weaned (largely by global food giant Kraft) onto processed cheese.

There is, nonetheless, a huge overlap between the Standard American Diet (SAD) and the consumption habits of the UK consumer. It is therefore legitimate to talk of the SO-BAD (the Standard Obese British-American Diet). How we, as a nation, can wean ourselves off the SO-BAD is the focal point of this book. Whether or not we succeed in doing so is arguably the biggest social and economic challenge we face over the coming decades. I firmly believe in the principle of individual responsibility as the key factor that will drive the necessary change. But for individuals to take action they need the right information and the right incentives. Alongside the individual there have been two other protagonists in the creation and exacerbation of this crisis: the government and the food industry itself. Neither of these, for differing reasons that I will explain, can be trusted to solve the obesity crisis.

Chapter 2: Movers & Shakers in the UK Grocery industry

"It is not the creation of wealth that is wrong, but the love of money for its own sake." Margaret Thatcher

In the United Kingdom, the food industry is extensive. It employs over 450,000 people and has a turnover in excess of £100bn. It is the largest manufacturing sector in the UK representing around 19% of total UK manufacturing output [1]. Worldwide processed food & drink sales exceed US$3 trillion and when we look at obesity it is the excessive processing of food that is the root cause of the problem. In high-level terms, processing food involves taking raw materials and adding either sugar, salt or fat (or a combination of all three) to create products that are then packed and shipped to our supermarkets where we put them in our shopping baskets.

The processed food industry is dominated by a few global players: Nestlé, Unilever, Kraft-Heinz,

PepsiCo, Coca Cola, General Mills, Mars, Mondelez, Kellogg's. Some of these companies have been around for over a century. All of them use highly sophisticated manufacturing, distribution, selling and marketing processes and techniques to sustain their success and drive profits. With the exception of the privately owned Mars Corporation, all of them are publicly quoted companies and thus obsessed with 'creating shareholder value', or more prosaically, 'making as much money as possible'. Despite what they may claim, they are not incentivised to solve the obesity crisis. I wouldn't go as far as saying that they don't care at all about our bulging waist-lines, it's just that when there's a trade-off between doing something about obesity and making more money to satisfy their demanding investors, it's no contest.

The reason I mention this is twofold. Firstly, we cannot expect the food industry to take the lead in addressing obesity. The government has, as you will learn shortly, tried, and failed, to engage the food companies in the obesity debate. Alcoholics don't vote for prohibition. Secondly, processed food, the major contributor to obesity, is engineered to precise specifications, often involving addictive amounts of sugar, fat and salt that make the end-product literally irresistible to the human palate. These products are then advertised, marketed, and promoted using techniques that are designed to maximise consumption, not optimise your and my calorie intake. As consumers we need to be aware of the tricks and deceptions that lead to over-consumption of the wrong foods and a consequent imbalance in our diet. Later in this book I will take you through the 'killer categories' that are the major contributors to the SO-BAD and point out how the brand owners, sometimes subtly, sometimes blatantly, but always knowingly, try to get you to eat more of their, often very fattening, highly addictive products.

One of the striking things about the global food industry is the influence of the big US corporations. Whilst Nestlé and Unilever fly the European flag, the rest of the big boys are all from the good old USA, which, as we now know, is the most obese major nation on earth. Coincidence?

Hardly. Alongside the big manufacturing giants there is another key group embroiled in the obesity epidemic: the big supermarkets. In the UK there is effectively an oligopoly of four major players controlling over 80% of grocery shopping: Tesco, Sainsbury's, Asda & Morrisons (latterly the German discounters Aldi & Lidl have started to gain a foothold). Their principal role is to distribute the products of their suppliers so in that respect they could legitimately argue that they are no more than middlemen in the interaction between consumers and manufacturers. Increasingly, however, the Big Four are becoming quasi-manufactures themselves as they expand their offer of own-label products that are often just cheaper versions of the big brands. Morrisons even owns some production facilities, making it the only one of the large grocery retailers to be truly vertically integrated. All of them, however, have a huge influence on their key own-label suppliers, sometimes to the extent that whole factories are dedicated to one key retailer.

In many food categories the copycat own brand version is not surprisingly, just as unhealthy and fattening as the brand leader (e.g. Sainsbury's Choco Rice Pops contain more sugar than Kellogg's Coco Pops). It would therefore be unfair to single out the food manufacturers as the only ones pedalling unhealthy products. The big retailers are also heavily implicated. The other key intervention of the retailers in our over-consumption of sugary, fatty processed food and drink is the deep-discounted promotion policy that they drive in conjunction with the big food manufacturers and their own own-label suppliers. Buy-one-get-one-free (or "BOGOF") is a common technique used indiscriminately for getting consumers to stock up on groceries.

In the last few years, we have also seen a rapid growth in out of home consumption and the related rise of home delivery services. An increasing part of the UK food industry is focused on food service and non-grocery in response to the changing consumption habits of UK consumers (particularly time-poor Millennials). Quick Serve Restaurants (QSR) such as

McDonalds, Nando's, KFC & Subway have expanded rapidly across the country. Chains such as Pret, Greggs, Eat and the numerous coffee shop franchises have significantly impacted our eating and drinking habits. This book is, however, primarily focused on grocery shopping (i.e. supermarkets). The rise of out of home consumption may well form the subject matter for the sequel to this book.

Within UK grocery, the last twenty years has seen one clear winner: Tesco. Founded at the end of the First World War by Jack Cohen who set up a market stall in Hackney, Tesco is now a truly global retail giant with 6,720 stores in eight different countries employing 450,000 people, with sales of £57bn and profits of over £2bn [2]. Cohen's famous quote of "pile it high, sell it cheap" has long since been replaced by "every little helps" but the relentless focus on value for money helped Tesco overtake Sainsbury's in 1995 to become the UK's largest supermarket. It now controls about 27% of the market, with Sainsbury's and Asda about half that share. No supplier (food manufacturer) has anything like the dominance of Tesco and it's fair to say that where Tesco have led in the last 30 years many of the others have followed: promotions, loyalty cards, pricing, store format, own-label ranging.

One of the key consequences of the emergence of the Tesco behemoth has been the growth of supermarket own-label products at the expense of manufacturer brands. In some categories (e.g. chilled foods) private label share is in excess of 60% and the chilled food manufacturers will often dedicate entire factories to one major retailer. In other categories, who actually makes the own-label product is often deliberately unclear. Some branded manufacturers will often produce retailer-branded products alongside their own. Others prefer to focus on their own brands and avoid potential conflicts of interest. Either way, Tesco and the other retailers do not have a problem finding suppliers eager to access their abundant distribution points. Crucially it is the retailer who determines the product specification of their own-label range – not the manufacturer, although they will be heavily involved in the process. Aldi & Lidl, the notoriously secretive German discounters, have contracts with many well-known branded goods manufacturers who would not like it made public that they supply these retailers with own-label at prices significantly below the price of their branded products for similar quality.

It almost goes without saying that the supplier side is far less consolidated and more fragmented than the retailer side where economies of scale are crucial. Nonetheless, scale and brand power are also important for suppliers as they constantly fight to keep their share of the profit pool that over the last few years has transferred to the retailers. According to the latest Forbes research, Nestlé is the world's largest food company by value with operations across a number of key categories including chocolate, coffee, dairy, water and pet food. The bulk of Nestlé's sales will go through big supermarket chains like Tesco, as will those of other Multinational Corporations (MNCs) like Unilever and Mars. Negotiations between MNCs and global retailers like Tesco involve multi-million pound sums to cover promotions, in-store activity, new product listings, on-line advertising etc. etc.

As the balance of power has shifted more towards retailers, manufacturers like Nestlé have sought out different routes to market, e.g. with Nespresso coffee going direct to consumer (DTC). For the time being however, they remain heavily reliant on the footfall that retailers generate through their bricks and mortar stores. The recent coronavirus crisis emphasised how important bricks & mortar supermarkets remain, despite the recent growth in on-line ordering and home delivery.

Every supermarket stocks tens of thousands of products and has commercial relationships with hundreds of suppliers from the MNCs like Nestlé to small local producers of sausages, cheese or beer. Slow-selling or unprofitable lines are quickly culled so there is a regular churn of products that are on the shelves. Maintaining rate of sale (ROS) and profit per unit are crucial for suppliers to keep their listings. In this cutthroat environment the retailers actively encourage suppliers to run promotions (e.g. multi-buy or discounts off the regular price). Tesco wants its average basket of good to be cheaper than any other retailers and will actively monitor prices across its competition, and pressure suppliers to give better terms. Supplying the major supermarkets is not for the faint-hearted as they will demand outstanding service levels and highly competitive prices. If as a supplier you can secure listings for your products you will, however, guarantee access to millions of shoppers and the opportunity to keep your factory full with regular orders.

The role of government & other industry bodies

The main government body overseeing the food industry in the UK is the Food Standards Agency (FSA). The following is taken from the FSA's own website:

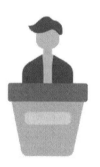

'The Food Standards Agency is responsible for food safety and food

hygiene in England, Wales and Northern Ireland. It works with local authorities to enforce food safety regulations and its staff work in meat plants to check the standards are being met.

The FSA also has responsibility for labelling policy in Wales and Northern Ireland, and for nutrition policy in Northern Ireland.'

In recent times the FSA has launched a number of high-profile initiatives designed to get people to make better choices about the food they consume. These include a campaign on salt reduction and a controversial traffic-light labelling initiative to which a number of manufacturers (and retailers) objected because they didn't like their products carrying a warning red mark indicating high levels of fat, sugar or salt.

After targeting salt, the FSA now has sugar firmly in its sights. In April 2018, the government introduced a new levy on sugary drinks, which are seen as a key driver of childhood obesity. Not surprisingly this tax was heavily contested by the likes of Coca Cola and Pepsi. A standard 330ml can of Coke contains 35g of sugar or about 7 teaspoons. Yet Coca Cola still defends its formulation and put the full weight of its legal team and PR department behind trying to prevent the so-called 'sugar tax'. The Food and Drink Federation (FDF), the voice of the UK food and drink industry, also came out in support of Coca Cola and the other drinks producers in fighting the tax.

I highlight this to illustrate how difficult it is for the government to legislate to help improve our diet. There are so many vested interests, which put profit before the general well-being of society. Another key government body is Public Health England, which lists amongst several key objectives, the following:

- making the public healthier and reducing differences between the health of different groups by promoting healthier lifestyles, advising government and supporting action by local government, the NHS and the public
- improving the health of the whole population by sharing our information and

expertise, and identifying and preparing for future public health challenges

- researching, collecting and analysing data to improve our understanding of public health challenges, and come up with answers to public health problems

One of PHE's more high-profile publications is its 'Eatwell Guide':

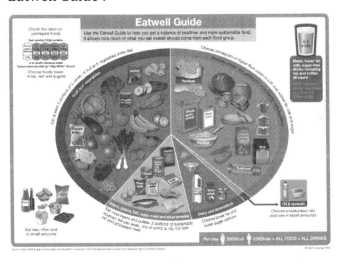

The above guidelines may have been produced by PHE, but lobbying from the food industry heavily influenced them. Whilst I would agree with some of the guidelines, a few of them require further scrutiny and challenge (e.g. the emphasis on grains and carbohydrates and the obsession with 5-a-day) of which more later.

Summary

The UK food industry is large and complex with a variety of key players and stakeholders. Many of our retailers, like Tesco, are truly world-class operators with seamless just-in-time supply chains and stores offering fantastic choice, quality, and value. Supermarkets partner with a whole range of suppliers from the 900lb gorillas like Nestlé with state-of-the-art factories to small artisanal producers. The government ensures the food we eat is safe and correctly labelled largely through the efforts of the FSA. As consumers we are now offered more choice and better value than at any time in human history. Unfortunately, we are increasingly making the wrong choices. The next chapter explores how and why we are encouraged to do so.

Chapter 3: The Marketing of Food

"Always look for the fool in the deal. If you don't find one, it's you." Mark Cuban

In the 1980s and 90s Procter & Gamble (P&G) established a reputation as arguably the leading consumer goods company on the planet, employing some of the brightest and best marketing talent. They had a fierce rivalry with Unilever in a number of categories including laundry & cleaning and personal care products but did not have Unilever's large footprint in food. P&G's ambition was to dominate the shopping basket, i.e. to get shoppers to fill up their basket with P&G brands. To achieve this goal, they would need to penetrate some of the big food categories like soft drinks.

When P&G enter a market, they tend to do it properly, with a fully resourced marketing plan that will give the launch the best chance of success. In April 1998 they invested £10million behind the launch of orange juice drink Sunny

Delight in the UK. The product was sold in refrigerated cabinets and marketed as a healthy alternative to soft drinks like Coke and Pepsi. Within 18 months Sunny Delight had remarkably become the third biggest selling drink in the UK behind the two cola giants. P&G had seemingly pulled off a huge success against the odds; entering an established market and rapidly taking share away from well-entrenched competitors.

The success didn't last, however, as the truth behind the marketing spin quickly emerged. Far from being healthy, Sunny Delight's main ingredient was high fructose corn syrup (HFCS) which is used by food and drinks manufacturers as a cheap alternative to cane sugar. Many experts consider HFCS to be a major driver of today's obesity epidemic [1]. The drink also only contained a small percentage of real fruit juice. It also didn't need to be kept in the fridge. Sunny Delight is an ambient product, but P&G knew that if people kept it in the fridge, they would drink more of it. When a story came out in the tabloid press of a young girl turning orange from drinking too much Sunny Delight, the game was up, and sales collapsed. P&G eventually sold the brand and ultimately gave up any ambitions to build a presence in food. The company is now focused entirely on non-food categories like health & beauty, where bold marketing claims are harder to contradict.

The above example illustrates the lengths that even normally ethical, well-respected companies like P&G will go to in their pursuit of sales and profits. In the case of Sunny Delight, the truth ultimately came out but, in the marketing of food, that is by no means always the case. It would be virtually impossible to cover all the tools and techniques that food companies and retailers use to get you, the consumer, to buy their products. In this chapter I will, however, try to highlight some of the more common ones so that next time you go shopping at least you will be armed with more information and less likely to be duped by some of the misleading marketing.

Marketers (and I know because I used to be one) love to talk about the 4 Ps: product, place, price & promotion. These are essentially the levers, or marketing mix, at their disposal to raise awareness of their product and to get you to buy it. At P&G they like to talk about the two moments of truth: in-store and at home. Winning these two moments is crucial to a brand's success: in-store the shopper is faced with a bewildering array of choices (an average supermarket has 50,000 stock-keeping units or SKUs). If the shopper doesn't put your product in their trolley, then they'll never get to the second moment of truth: consuming the product at home.

So as well as having a great product (or at the very least a product that will get bought again once consumed) the marketing department has to grab the shopper's attention in store through packaging, pricing, promotions and other means. If, like me, you are a child of the sixties, you'll recall that in the 70s and 80s TV advertising was dominated by food brands: Beanz Meanz Heinz, For Mash get Smash (an instant mash potato!), A Mars a Day, I'd like to buy the world a Coke, etc. These were iconic adverts that drove huge sales in the good old days when there was less competition and the balance of power was still with suppliers rather than retailers. In recent times marketing a food brand has become much more difficult and marketers are far less dependent on TV campaigns, although they still play a role.

Product (& packaging)

Let's go through the key elements of the marketing mix to highlight the way marketers seek to successfully influence consumers in the food aisles on their weekly shop. Products and packaging come in all shapes and sizes. As already mentioned, food labelling and ingredients listing is strictly controlled by the FSA, but this does not stop food companies pushing the boundaries. The 'traffic-light' system was fiercely contested by both retailers (some not all) and suppliers before being finally mandated by the FSA in 2013.

One of the most common tricks is the 'low-fat' claim which was especially prevalent 5-10 years ago when fat was being demonised and we were all being encouraged to reduce fat in our diet. The flip side of this claim is usually high sugar, so I guess you have to decide which you feel is worse. I will cover a little about dieting later on but let's just say for now there is compelling evidence that too much sugar and not too much fat is driving obesity [2]. Also, sugar (in its many and varied forms) is cheap and plentiful, so which ingredient do you think food companies would rather sell?

The other claim that has grown in popularity in recent years is 'natural' which food marketers know through their focus groups and other research methodologies is a word with strong appeal to consumers. It basically gives people the assurance that there is nothing harmful in their food and that it is as good as they could make at home without the hassle of preparing it themselves. Unfortunately, it is not quite as straightforward as it may seem. Additives, particularly E-numbers, are badly perceived but play an important role in food production as stabilisers, preservatives, and flavour enhancers. The drive towards 'clean labelling', i.e. only ingredients that you would have in your own kitchen, has driven food companies to seek natural replacements for some of the scarier sounding chemicals in their recipes. As a rule of thumb, the more processed the food, the longer the ingredients list. And the longer the ingredients list, the more you should be wary. Don't be fooled by 'low-fat', natural or other seductive claims. Read the ingredient list and make your own judgement.

For example, take a look at McVitie's Go Ahead! Yoghurt Breaks, Forest Fruit biscuits. The packaging describes them as a 'delicious yogurt flavour topping on a light crispy biscuit with a sultana and berry flavoured filling'. The ingredient list is as long as your arm and includes: a baking agent (maltitol syrup), humectant (glycerine), sodium and ammonium bicarbonate, calcium carbonate, E472e, disodium diphosphate and a stabiliser (calcium lactate). Colourful pictures of juicy forest fruits feature prominently on the packaging, but we are told in small print that the product contains the equivalent of 0.2% of raspberries, strawberries, redcurrants and blackberries. One fifth of one per cent! If you are looking for fruit, then you should look elsewhere, but the packaging would have you believe it was bursting with freshly picked berries.

Food manufacturers are also good at picking up on the latest fads and trends. Protein is currently on trend as low-carb/high-protein diets grow in popularity. A word of caution, however, for products (particularly snack bars) labelled "high protein". Very often these products are high in sugar so if you are following a low-carb diet they will not help.

Similarly, vegetarianism and veganism are currently resurgent. I am personally a meat-eater but can understand and empathise with the motives of vegans and vegetarians and I do sometimes eat meat-free meals. Unfortunately, the food industry is exploiting the meat-free trend by unnecessarily labelling a lot of fundamentally unhealthy processed products as suitable for vegans/vegetarians.

Can you guess which product this is?:

Mycoprotein (92%), Rehydrated Free Range Egg White, Natural Caramelised Sugar, Firming Agents: Calcium Chloride, Calcium Acetate; Gluten Free Barley Malt Extract

It reads like a chemistry experiment, but it is actually the ingredient list for the market leading meat-alternative brand Quorn. I understand and empathise with those people who are vegetarian for environmental, ethical, and animal welfare reasons but is this really the best alternative? In the next chapter I will continue this theme when I look at some of the biggest categories and biggest selling brands in our supermarkets but for the time being, heed the message: don't be fooled by the what the packaging says! If you don't recognise many of the ingredients, then don't buy it.

Place

The next of the 'Four Ps' of marketing is place or, in other words, the distribution, ranging and merchandising of the product. Coca Cola famously has the mantra of always having its drinks 'within an arm's length of desire'. The task of food companies is not simply getting their product listed in the major supermarket, it is crucial to get the right number of facings in the right place in the shelf. The ideal spot is at about shoulder height, directly in the eye-line of the shopper, and multiple-facings of the same product have been proven to drive increased sales. Food manufacturers have sophisticated 'category management' teams who are tasked with working with retailers to optimise the shelf layouts to drive rate of sale (ROS) and profit per square foot. The most profitable lines survive, the rest are ruthlessly culled. So, although you have plenty of choice when you go to the supermarket, you will be subconsciously encouraged to put those items in your basket that maximise the profits of the retailer.

Price

The third 'P' in the marketing mix is price, which is less straightforward than you might at first think. Manufacturers often take a cost-plus approach to pricing where they take the costs of production and give themselves an acceptable level of gross margin to work out the selling price to the supermarket. The supermarket then adds on their margin to come up with a Recommended Selling Price (RSP) to you, the shopper. The big 4 UK supermarkets are obsessed with relative pricing. Tesco does not want Sainsbury's or Asda selling a product cheaper and vice-versa. This is good news in one respect for shoppers as this intense competition helps drive down prices. The corollary of this is that suppliers are driven to constantly make things cheaper. Reformulating, or to use the industry jargon, 're-engineering', products is a constant focus. Swapping out expensive ingredients for cheaper ones is a daily focus for food companies with teams of development chefs and product developers engaged in the process: an ice-cream manufacturer might swap cream or milk for vegetable oil, a bakery might use margarine instead of butter in its croissants, the cod in fish fingers is replaced with farmed fish, the jar of maple syrup is no longer 100% maple syrup and is now a hybrid containing other sweeteners, the chicken on the rotisserie was battery farmed, your favourite strawberry jam is more sugar than strawberries.

The price of our average basket of groceries has tumbled in real teams over the last 40 years, but at what cost to our health? Decades of 'reengineering' have brought prices down but have resulted in bastardised versions of many of our household staples. In an era where we spend hundreds of pounds on mobile phones and Netflix subscriptions, are we no longer willing to pay for quality food? Or are we just unaware of the gradual erosion of our food values?

In his school meals campaign, Jamie Oliver did an excellent job of killing off the Turkey Twizzler, made from mechanically recovered meat, but even he can't police every food crime in every supermarket. The food industry would, with some justification, argue that there is extensive choice and that consumers always have healthy options available. So why are we becoming fatter as a nation? Why is life expectancy reducing in some parts of the UK for the first time in living memory? The affordability of many highly processed, low-quality foods is surely a factor, as is the increasing desire for convenience amongst shoppers. A healthier diet is arguably no more expensive than an unhealthy one and later on I will show you ways to save money on several key items in your weekly shop.

Promotion

The final 'P' is promotion, which covers a range of activities from temporary price reductions to multi-buy offers through to brand advertising. In-store promotions are many and varied. They include the controversial 'Buy One Get One Free' (BOGOF) deal, which encourages shoppers to load their pantry with products at half price but also potentially encourages over-consumption and increased food waste. There are watered down versions of the BOGOF deal, e.g. Buy One Get Second Half Price, or 3 for the price of 2, but in nearly all cases the promotion is heavily funded by the manufacturer rather than the retailer. Why does this matter? Food manufacturers know that the marginal cost of producing a few more products on their production lines is much less than the standard or average cost. Running the factory for a little longer to produce extra volume for a promotion and can be justified on economic grounds by the accountants. Over time, however, shoppers get used to promotions and do not like paying full price anymore. The retailer will sometimes actively encourage this behaviour. They want loyalty to their supermarket not to manufacturers. So, if Brand X runs a promotion one week, Brand Y might run one the following week. The shopper, as long as they are indifferent to Brands X & Y, gets two weeks of great deals. Pantry-loading promotions like these are often run by the biggest food processors that have the deepest pockets. They also tend to sell some of the unhealthiest products. Well, I suppose a BOGOF on lentils will not excite too many people compared to one on Jaffa Cakes.

Promotional budgets for big brands can run into millions of pounds and for retailers can be a huge source of additional profits. Tesco became embroiled in an accounting scandal a few years ago when it was found to be overstating its profits by up to £250m, in part because of the way it handled accounting for promotions with suppliers. Both retailers and suppliers are to some extent hooked on the promotional 'drug' as an important lever in driving sales and profits.

Outside of the supermarket, food brands will seek to raise awareness for their products through more traditional promotional methods such as advertising. Gone are the days when ITV had a virtual monopoly on TV advertising. There are many different TV channels these days alongside the burgeoning social media platforms. Your favourite crisp brand is just as likely to pop up on Facebook as during the ad-break in Coronation Street. In an ideal world for the food marketer you will see the advertising, put the product on your shopping list and go into the supermarket to buy it. Once you have consumed it you will hopefully continue to buy every week. The big dirty secret of many brands is that they rely on so-called 'heavy users' of their products. My former employer, Mars, long ago ditched the slogan 'a Mars a day helps you work rest and play' but they know that many people do eat at least one bar of chocolate a day, contrary to all healthy eating guidelines. A standard 'meal-deal' in many convenience stores consists of a sandwich and a bag of crisps. As a nation we consume more crisps per head than virtually anywhere else on the planet, but you don't hear the executives at Walkers urging people to exercise restraint. On the contrary, they have one of the most active marketing campaigns in the industry, making their brand worth nearly £1 billion for owners PepsiCo.

The food industry loves to promote the 'calories-in/calories-out' theory of consumption. The hypothesis they would like you to buy into is that there is no such thing as bad foods and that if you exercise enough then you won't get fat. The truth is, **you can't outrun a bad diet**. You only need to take a look at the list of the UK's top food brands and you begin to understand why we are becoming more and more unhealthy as a nation:

1. Cadbury's, retail sales value £1.7bn
2. Coca Cola £1.4bn
3. Nestlé £1.1bn
4. Walkers £1bn

5. Heinz £0.6bn

All of the above brands belong to powerful multi-national corporations (MNCs) with huge financial resources using highly sophisticated sales and marketing techniques. They are relentless in driving value for their shareholders and maximising market share but less interested in your wellbeing. I recall one conversation with a board member of Heinz when I worked there responsible for marketing beans. Branston had just launched a range of baked beans to compete with Heinz's market leader. "Can't we just stick a hose down their neck and drown the f*****?" was the helpful advice I received to eliminate our new unwelcome competition. Heinz Baked Beans and Ketchup are extremely high in salt and sugar, but Heinz are reluctant to change the recipes, as they know what works. Admittedly they have launched low-sugar and low-salt versions of their brands, but these are not marketed with anything like the resources of the bestsellers.

Walkers has the muscle of PepsiCo behind it and has successfully used ex-footballer turned TV presenter Gary Lineker in one of the longest-running marketing campaigns ever seen in the UK. Lineker tends to get very defensive when asked about his promotion of junk food, unusually so for someone so outspoken on other ethical and moral issues of our time. At 3.5kg/head/year the humble potato crisp is Britain's favourite savoury snack (only the Irish eat more globally). High in salt and saturated fat, crisps also contain acrylamide as a by-product of the high temperature cooking process. Acrylamide is considered a dangerous carcinogen. In a 2017 study, one in five potato crisp varieties were found to have acrylamide above the recommended level [3]. Supermarket own brand products performed worse than major snack brands like Walkers, but all fried crisps contain some traces of the cancer-causing chemical. You won't find any mention of this in the marketing but the European Food Safety Authority (EFSA) confirms that 'acrylamide levels in food have the potential to increase the risk of cancer for people of all ages'. Our own FSA states that 'it's not possible to establish a safe level of exposure for acrylamide'. Next time the avuncular Lineker encourages you to eat more crisps, tell him to stick to football.

Number 2 on the list needs no introduction. There have been numerous books charting the remarkable story of Coca Cola, arguably one of the world's first truly global brands. Less well known is the aggressive way they have defended their territory with their formidable legal resources and PR machine. They were heavily behind a lot of research in the 1970s and 80s defending sugar and demonising fat. More recently they were still pushing the calories out argument and pinning rising obesity on people's sedentary lifestyles. They furiously fought the introduction of the sugar tax on soft drinks and persuaded the FDF and other influential bodies to speak out on their behalf. There are of course zero sugar and low sugar versions of their leading brands, but the latest research on artificial sweeteners, which these versions contain, doesn't make great reading if you care remotely about what you put in your body. (See Chapter 4, Carbonated Soft Drinks for more detail on the negative effects of artificial sweeteners).

Nestlé Food (excluding coffee) derives its £1bn plus sales from a combination of its established chocolate brands (Kit Kat, Yorkie, Rolo, etc.), sugary cereals (Shreddies, Cheerios, etc.), and its Buitoni pasta brand. Based out of Switzerland it expanded its UK business through the acquisition of York-based chocolate maker Rowntree's in 1988 and has a joint venture with General Mills in breakfast cereals. It also sells yoghurts under a variety of brand names, most with added sugar.

Cadbury is the largest food brand in the UK, and with its iconic purple packaging and familiar logo it has a rich history. Its founder, John Cadbury, was a philanthropic Quaker who built a town, Bourneville, for his workers. At the time of writing, Cadbury is launching a new campaign in the UK to celebrate Easter. According to its marketing team; "We see Easter as a holiday to reawaken the generous spirit in people; a Cadbury Easter egg is all it takes to connect with your loved ones and show you care."

Cadbury is now owned by Mondelez. Last year in the UK the company generated £1.7billion in revenues and profits of £35 million. The company paid a grand total of £271,000 in tax. Maybe Cadbury could show how much it cares by paying a bit more tax? With Type 2 diabetes on the rise the NHS is going to need even more resources. Cadbury is an advocate of the calories out philosophy. A few years ago, it ran a much-criticised promotional campaign whereby kids could get vouchers for school sports equipment by buying its chocolate bars. Just to get a basketball required buying 170 bars, which takes 90 hours of exercise to burn off. After much adverse publicity, the promotion was dropped.

One of Cadbury's iconic Easter products is the famous Crème Egg. A 40g Crème Egg contains 26.5g of sugar. Let that sink it: two thirds of a Crème Egg is pure sugar! Now I do not want to sound like a killjoy. I love a bit of chocolate as much as the next man, but we eat far too much in this country (at 7.6kg/head p.a. almost twice as much as France) and it is literally killing us.

Summary

Food is a multi-billion pound industry. We spend around £200bn every year in our supermarkets. The most lucrative products for the suppliers and retailers tend to be the more processed and unhealthy ones. A bar of chocolate has a higher profit margin than an apple. The 900lb gorillas in the food jungle are the MNCs who have world-class production facilities that churn out standardised products at an optimised cost. Over the years they have re-engineered recipes to make their brands even more profitable and, in many cases, more unhealthy. Food is distributed through world-class supply chains that ensure optimum availability and choice for supermarket shoppers.

It is true that if you want to buy healthily you can, even if this might at times cost a little more. The fact is many of us are not making the right choices. The big brands dominate with share of shelf as well as share of mind. Through a potent mix of creative advertising, attractive packaging, distribution, slick category management, merchandising, and in-store promotions, the largest food companies reinforce their dominant market position through increased sales.

The five biggest brands in the UK are all essentially junk (either high sugar, high salt, additive-heavy, overly processed or a combination of everything). They should only be eaten occasionally - even PHE agree with me on this - and should not be part of a daily food regime. The reason they form the top 5 is that many people consume them far too much, far too often. Heavy-users (often in both senses of the term!) are a food-marketers dream customer: the person who starts his day with a bowl of sugary cereal, treats himself to a bar of chocolate daily, always has a packet of crisps with his lunchtime sandwich, puts ketchup on everything and washes it down with a regular fizzy soft drink. Our habits need to change if we are going to halt the obesity epidemic but do not expect the food industry giants to help drive that change. They are too busy making money while you get ill.

Chapter 4: The Killer Categories

"Don't use a knife and fork to dig your own grave"
Anon.

In this section I will cover the food categories, which I believe are having the biggest impact on obesity and negatively impacting our health. I should stress that I will not be covering tobacco or alcohol as both are strictly regulated and their effect on public health has been well documented and communicated. Instead I will be focusing on the processed foods that have become staples for many shoppers, shedding some light on how they are produced and the consequences of regular and frequent consumption. By the end of this section you will know a lot more about the food you buy, how it is made, what is in it, and how often (if ever) you should consume it. I will highlight the market leaders in each category so you can see who is behind the brand. And to help you shop better I will grade each category with a shopping trolley key:

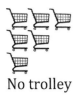 Can form part of your weekly shop
Every now and again
Very occasional purchase
No trolley   Leave on the shelf

Breakfast Cereals

Let's start appropriately enough with the first meal of the day. Back in 1876 Dr John Harvey Kellogg was running a sanatorium in Battle Creek, Michigan with 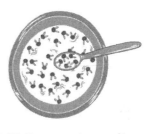 the help of his brother, W.K. Kellogg. According to popular myth, the good doctor hit upon the recipe for corn flakes while he was trying to find a 'cure' for masturbation! Spoiler alert: it didn't work, but they did by chance hit upon a recipe for the first Corn Flakes. The two brothers ultimately fell out and W.K. Kellogg went on to launch the Battle Creek Toasted Corn Flake Company. The foundations of a global business had been laid and Kellogg's is to this day the biggest breakfast cereal producer in the world with global sales of over £10bn and £0.5bn in the UK alone, making it the UK's 10th biggest food brand.

The original Corn Flakes were, given their origins, developed as a health food but the current Kellogg's range has strayed a long way from its medicinal roots. It did not take W.K. Kellogg long to work out that adding sugar to his products improved taste and resulted in higher sales. Fast forward about 100 years and their portfolio of brands today, alongside the iconic Corn Flakes, includes Frosties, Coco Pops, Rice Krispies, Crunchy Nut, Special K, Krave, and the virtuous sounding Just Right.

According to PHE Chief Executive, Duncan Selbie "Kids consume half their daily sugar allowance before the school bell rings, with much of it coming from cereals." In 2017, Kellogg's finally bowed to pressure from the sugar lobby and agreed to axe its Ricicles brand and reduce the sugar content of some of its other kids' brands like Coco Pops by as much as 40%. It also agreed to stop marketing Frosties to kids admitting that the majority of consumption was by adults. These changes were long overdue and arguably too little, too late. Frosties still contains 37% sugar, Crunchy Nut 35% and the ironically named Just Right a whopping 23%. After several years of decline in the UK, Kellogg's finally got back to growth in 2019, largely thanks to increased sales of two of its sweetest offerings: Frosties and Crunchy Nut. "This is Crunchy Nut's third consecutive year of growth, which shows shoppers still value taste within their breakfast choices," said a Kellogg's spokesperson in an interview with The Grocer magazine. Well I suppose that is one way of looking at it. Another take on it might be that after spending years and millions of pounds getting people addicted to sugar, then guess what, they're still addicted!

Nestlé (through its partnership with General Mills) is the other big branded player in breakfast cereals with Cheerios, Shreddies, Shredded Wheat and Golden Grahams amongst its best sellers. The lowest sugar content of these is Shreddies at 13% rising to 25% for Golden Grahams. Standard Cheerios are 18% sugar with the honey variety at

22%. The reason the cereal manufacturers are reluctant to reduce sugar is that they know that it will negatively impact sales. Over the years they have attuned our taste buds to ever sweeter products and reformulating recipes is not only technically difficult, but it affects best before dates and potentially cost as sugar is cheap and plentiful.

There are, of course, low sugar and zero-added sugar cereals available in the supermarkets. Standard Weetabix at 4.2% is relatively low but some of the other variants like Weetabix Choc Chip minis are as high as 21%. You might think that the retailers, via their own brand products, would be more responsible. Sainsbury's Choc Rice Pops contains, however, 28% sugar, higher than the equivalent Kellogg's product.

My personal view is that anything above 5% sugar should not form part of a regular breakfast regime, which would effectively wipe out many of the leading brands from our supermarket shelves. There have been many studies highlighting the importance of breakfast, and in particular, of consuming foods with a low glycaemic index (GI) that help you feel fuller for longer. Porridge oats (zero added sugar!) are a good example as is the good old egg, the breakfast of choice for previous generations.

Trolley recommendation:

High sugar cereals > 5%
Porridge Oats, sugar free muesli

Bread

Back in the early 1980s one of my first temporary jobs was working on the delivery vans at the local Warburtons factory

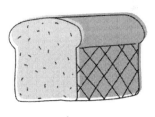

dropping off bread at various convenience stores. Warburtons has since expanded outside of its Lancashire heartland to become a truly national brand with sales of over £650m, making it the largest bread brand in the UK. Hovis, with sales of just under £300m and Kingsmill at £194m are the other big national players, which not surprisingly make bread one of the biggest categories in the grocery store.

Bread is of course a much-revered foodstuff that has been a staple food in many cultures throughout much of human history. According to history, the Egyptians in 800BC were the first people to make what we today recognise as chapatis or tortillas, a flatbread made from a simple paste of flour and water. Bread has evolved to be eaten in many different formats around the world. The French love their baguette, the Germans have a great variety of seeded loaves, rye and black bread, Middle Eastern and Asian cultures still prefer flatbreads. The Italian ciabatta was surprisingly only invented as recently as the 1980s. Here in the UK, however, we think the best thing is the sliced loaf and most sales come in that format. When I lived in France most people's daily routine involved a trip to the 'boulangerie' (baker) to buy fresh bread. Why daily? Well if you didn't eat it the same day it would go stale overnight because it doesn't contain any additives or preservatives.

The humble baguette is a simple classic that the French will not tamper with. Us Brits are a little more laissez-faire about our food and the primacy of the white sliced mass-produced loaf can be traced back to a small Hertfordshire village in the early 1960s.

In those early post-war years, scientists at the Chorleywood Flour Milling and Bakery Research Association developed a process for low protein British wheat that produced a 40% softer, uniform loaf that could be baked in a fraction of time versus the standard process. The flip side of this revolutionary way of baking was the addition of hard fats, extra yeast, emulsifiers, enzymes, and other chemicals. 'Fast' bread like fast food comes at a cost of being less natural and more industrially processed. Not for nothing is it known in the trade as 'plant bread' or factory bread. An artisan baker would not recognise this method of making our daily staple. Around 80% of the bread produced in Britain today is Chorleywood bread. Ironically, the process was originally developed to help smaller bakers compete with the big industrial giants, but the big players quickly adopted it themselves. As I have already highlighted, with Big Food, lower cost usually wins over higher quality.

Not surprisingly a cheap and plentiful product does not appear to be especially valued by consumers: one third of the bread bought in Britain every year (680,000 tonnes) is thrown away. Moreover, reported food intolerances and allergies linked to Chorleywood bread have risen dramatically in recent years. Artisanal breads, including sourdough, are staging a comeback as people begin to value again the simplicity of traditionally made loaves. Standard plant bread has seen some of the biggest declines of any major grocery category in recent years. To borrow a phrase attributed to Abraham Lincoln: "You can't fool all the people all of the time". I believe and hope that the public mood is turning against Chorleywood bread with its chemicals and preservatives. Kingsmill's sales are dropping like a stone, down over 17% (£40m) in a year. At Warburton's, bread no longer makes up the bulk of sales after successful expansion into other bakery categories like crumpets and bagels.

Hovis has been in steady decline for several years, despite bringing back its famous 'boy on the bike' TV advertising.

With bread, as with nearly all foods, simpler is better and people are beginning to change their habits. Unfortunately, the bread manufacturers are less keen to drive change. They have millions of pounds of fixed assets tied up in existing bakeries that churn out Chorleywood plant bread. Re-configuring factories is expensive and investing in new production processes in a declining bread market is like trying to catch a falling knife.

My optimistic view is that with the changing nature of our high streets we may see the return of the artisan baker like in France. Wouldn't it be great to see a return to daily fresh bread produced locally? And don't be fooled by the supermarkets' in-store bakeries. One food critic has dismissed them as nothing more than 'tanning salons' where frozen dough is 'baked off' to produce a wide variety of seemingly fresh products. The reality is that many of these products contain the same additives and chemicals as those sitting on the ambient shelves nearby. Astonishingly these in-store bakery products are not subject to the same ingredient labelling laws as on-shelf products, so it is not so easy for shoppers to see. Take care also with ready to eat, pre-packed sandwiches. They are nearly all made with Chorleywood plant bread and can be a major source of excess salt in your diet.

Trolley recommendation:

Chorleywood bread (i.e. most sliced supermarket loaves)

If you are a regular consumer of bread then seek out freshly made, zero additive versions made by an artisan baker. You will be amazed at the variety of breads on offer if you look outside the standard sliced loaves.

Non-dairy Spreads (Margarines)

Given we have been talking about bread it seems logical to talk about the stuff we put on it. Back in the days before the scientists at Chorleywood effectively  switched us all away from real bread, the topping of choice was of course butter and for many of us, it still is. Lurpak (Sales £342m) and Anchor (£121m) both sit in the list of top 100 brands. The first butter substitute was invented in France in 1869 and over time both the manufacturing and marketing of margarine has evolved dramatically. From being a cheap alternative to butter, margarine is now pushed as a healthier, plant-based option compared to the saturated-fat rich, single ingredient substance produced by cows.

Older readers will recall that back in the 80s and 90s, Unilever's market-leading Flora brand was sold as 'the margarine for men' as men, not women, had heart attacks so should avoid eating that nasty butter. Saturated fats were demonised then and continue to be touted as a source of high cholesterol and hence heart disease to this day. For what it's worth there have been a number of scientific studies, including one funded by the British Heart Foundation in 2014 involving 600,000 participants that found no link between saturated fat consumption and coronary heart disease.

For many years, margarine was produced with trans fats, which we now know to be seriously bad for you with a definitive link to heart disease. Back in 1993, market-leader Flora contained 21% trans fats while most other margarines were a third trans fats. Although trans fats are not officially banned in the UK, most manufacturers have taken steps in the last 10 years to remove them from their products. You may recall the fulsome apology from margarine producers for all those years of feeding us trans fats and giving the misleading impression that they were healthier than butter? No, you don't remember? That's because it never happened. Flora went on to have a long association with the London Marathon to try and cement its healthy image in consumers' minds. In her book Swallow This (Serving Up The Food Industry's Darkest Secrets), Joanna Blythman has this to say about margarine:

"(Margarine is) an edible construction that owes its very existence to technology. It is a forced marriage of two cheap substances that won't naturally come together: oil – refined and processed out of all recognition – and water. This unwilling twosome is coerced into an alliance brokered by emulsifying additives. The resulting slippery sludge then needs to be coloured to be lifted out of murky greyness, flavoured to help us get it down our gullets, fortified with vitamins it lacks, and spiked with substances to stop it turning rancid."

Does that sound like something you should be putting on your toast? The top brass at Unilever decided a couple of years ago that the margarine market was as unattractive as the product itself and sold their entire global spreads business to private equity giant KKR in a $8 billion deal. Last year the leading brand in the newly created

Upfield UK portfolio, Flora, had a double-digit decline (-10.5%) but is still worth some £115m and is the 75th biggest food brand in UK grocery. The marketing message has switched away from spurious heart health to emphasising the plant-based credentials of margarine: '100% Plant Goodness' screams the packaging. There is even a dairy-free vegan version in the range. Now call me a cynic but a carrot or an apple in their unadulterated form could legitimately claim to be '100% Plant Goodness' but not margarine produced as above.

Private Equity firms are not known for their long-term approaches to businesses they acquire and KKR will be looking to profitably exit from Upfield within the next 3-5 years. In the meantime, they aim to exploit the growing trend in vegetarianism and veganism by pushing their products as a legitimate plant-based alternative to butter. Butter has been around for thousands of years, is 100% natural, additive-free, with a demonstrably better taste than margarine. The bad science that has led to the demonization of saturated fats is gradually being proved wrong. I realise that certain groups of consumers, be it for ethical or allergy/intolerance reasons, do not want to eat butter. Margarine is not a credible alternative. Ironically 'I Can't Believe It's Not Butter' (or as I prefer to call it 'I Can't Believe It's Not Banned') is another leading brand in the Upfield portfolio. Margarine producers have been churning out poor imitations of butter for years. It is fools' gold – do your body, and your taste buds, a favour, don't buy it.

Trolley recommendation:

Margarine	Zero
Butter (ideally organic)	🛒🛒🛒

NB. A word of caution: there is 'hidden' margarine in many bakery products in the supermarket. A lot of cheaper pastry, biscuits and cakes are made with margarine rather than butter. If you are going to treat yourself to a Danish or croissant, go for the all-butter version if you can find it. Also 'spreadable butters' are often a hybrid of butter and margarine and should also be avoided.

Carbonated Soft Drinks (CSDs)

Fizzy soda is a staple of the Standard American Diet (SAD) and like most things American found its way to the UK in the post-war years. Apart from Coke there are several other CSDs in the UK's top 100 brands list including 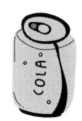 Coca Cola's arch-rival Pepsi, Fanta, Irn Bru (the preferred CSD of Scots), Dr. Pepper and energy drinks Red Bull and Monster. Selling sugar and water is seriously big business! The sales of just these brands listed above total over £2.6 billion in the UK. Drinking sugar and water is also potentially seriously damaging to your health if you are a regular and frequent consumer of CSDs. The following is taken from an article published in Medical News Today in January 2018:

'Researchers from multiple institutions across the globe, including the Special Institute for Preventive Cardiology and Nutrition in Salzburg, Austria, the Geneva University Hospitals in Switzerland, and the University of Navarra in

Spain, have teamed up to analyse recent studies targeting the potential link between sugary drinks and obesity.

"The evidence base linking Sugar Sweetened Beverages (SSBs) with obesity and overweight in children and adults has grown substantially in the past 3 years," says review co-author Dr. Nathalie Farpour-Lambert. "We were able to include 30 new studies not sponsored by the industry in this review, an average of 10 per year."

"Recent evidence suggests that SSB consumption is positively associated with obesity in children. By combining the already published evidence with this new research, we conclude [that] public health policies should aim to reduce the consumption of SSBs and encourage healthy alternatives such as water."

The researchers looked at 20 studies addressing the link between SSBs and obesity in children (17 prospective and three randomized controlled trials) as well as 10 studies investigating this link in the case of adults (nine prospective and one randomized controlled trial).

Of all the studies, 93% concluded that there was a "positive association" between the onset of overweight or obesity and the consumption of sugary drinks in both children and adults.

Just one prospective cohort study found no link between SSBs and excess weight in the case of children.'"

For years, the big soft drink brands have tried to argue that they are not, at least partially responsible, for the growing obesity crisis. Coca-Cola is still peddling the 'calories-out' argument on its website and fought tooth and nail against the sugar tax introduced in 2018 as did many others in the industry. They are swimming against the tide. The evidence that SSBs are a major causative factor in the increasing rates of obesity across the globe is becoming irrefutable.

The counter argument they often cite is that they also offer a range of low-calorie or zero-calorie drinks as part of their brand portfolio. It's true, Coke Zero, Pepsi Max, Diet Coke, reduced sugar Red Bull, etc., are all readily available and big sellers in their own right. But are they necessarily any healthier given they are loaded with artificial sweeteners? In 2013 a wide-ranging review of studies looking at the impact of such sweeteners on weight and other health outcomes came to this overall conclusion:

"Accumulating evidence suggests that frequent consumers of these sugar substitutes may also be at increased risk of excessive weight gain, metabolic syndrome, type-2 diabetes, and cardiovascular disease."

Not exactly a ringing endorsement for the diet version of your favourite fizzy drink is it? More worryingly, many of the sugar and high-fructose corn syrup (HFCS) alternatives are chemically synthesised sweeteners that are potentially dangerous if consumed in high quantities. Although currently not banned by health authorities despite their toxicity, investigative food journalist Joanna Blythman points out, "studies have linked artificial sweetener consumption to a variety of negative health effects: migraine, epilepsy, premature birth and brain cancer."

I do not want to completely denigrate CSDs but at the current levels of consumption they represent a major risk to public health. The marketing and PR machine behind the CSD industry is one of the biggest and best funded you will come across. Corporations like Coca-Cola and Pepsi aggressively defend their businesses, often sponsoring research to support their standpoint, lobbying governments and regulators, challenging and slowing down legislation (e.g. the sugar tax), and making specious claims, e.g. linking diet and lifestyle to shift the blame back onto their consumers. Along with multi-million-pound advertising budgets it's no surprise that people continue to buy CSDs in enormous quantities. It is not a fair fight and we are not given a balanced argument with the right level of transparency.

Encouragingly the first indications are that the sugar tax is working. Many drinks producers showed hitherto unseen speed in reformulating their offer to meet the new guidelines. Half of them have reformulated their drinks with lower sugar recipes to reduce the tax they pay (Coca Cola chose not to). Consequently, the expected tax revenue has fallen from £520m to an anticipated £240m in the first year. Opponents of the sugar tax argued strongly that it is a regressive tax. The reality is that obesity affects the poorest in our society and just because it is regressive does not mean that it is not effective. This was a long overdue initiative, which will save lives in the long run. Coca-Cola and their competitors will continue to complain but, as I have already said, they are motivated by profits and are not concerned with the health of the general public.

Trolley recommendation:

Coke, Pepsi or other CSD

Bottled Water

So, if, as I recommend, you give CSDs a swerve, what should you drink to quench your thirst and stay hydrated? We are fortunate to live in the UK, a first world country with a temperate climate and access to virtually free, clean running water. When I was growing up 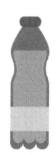 in Lancashire my old Dad used to call it 'Corporation Pop' and, although I did not appreciate it at the time, there is no better drink. It has zero calories and if you drink too much your body will easily deal with the excess. Most of us drink too little not too much.

If you had told me as a child that people would pay for water in plastic bottles, I wouldn't have believed you. So how did it come about that we started to spend so much money on a beverage that is virtually free and almost universally accessible? Clearly a big factor is lifestyle change. Eating and drinking on the go is no longer socially unacceptable and bottled water is now as ubiquitous as Coke. If you look at the list of the top 100 UK grocery brands, four of them are bottled water. Volvic (Sales £169m), Evian (£155m), Highland Spring (£125m), Buxton (£110m) are the major players in a category that is finally slowing down in the UK after years of stellar growth. Globally, however, the industry is estimated to be worth a staggering $100billion. Volvic and Evian are both owned by large French food corporation Danone and are imported into the UK from France. Yes, our rainy country with an abundant supply of clean drinking water, ships in lorry loads of plastic bottles of water from across the channel every month. At least Nestlé-owned Buxton can claim to be British, emanating from the eponymous spa town in the Peak district.

The environmental impact of bottled water is the real thorny issue. It is not the product per se, it's the packaging. It takes around 1.32 litres of water to make 1 litre of bottled water. An estimated 80% of plastic water bottles end up in landfill. Add to that the transportation impact of shipping water around nationally and internationally. There should be more water fountains available in public places and major transport hubs like railway stations and airports to encourage people to use refillable bottles. From a nutritional and health standpoint there is nothing wrong with bottled water. Some people claim it tastes better than tap water. In the past I have done some crude blind tests and the results seem to indicate that in reality people can't tell the difference. If, as we all should, you care about the environmental impact then, where possible, choose good old Corporation Pop over plastic bottles. You know it makes sense! It is estimated that bottled water is 1,000 times more expensive than tap water so think of all the money you're saving while helping the planet.

Trolley recommendation: only if you have no access to running water

Yoghurts

When I was a child growing up in the seventies, yoghurts were not a mainstream product in the British diet. The pioneer was a brand called Ski, since acquired by Nestlé, which promised 'that sunny morning feeling' in its advertising. It was the first yoghurt with added fruit and sugar to appear on the UK market and paved the way for a huge explosion in the category. Müller is today the market leader with sales of just under £500m making it the ninth biggest brand in UK grocery. Yoghurt has traditionally had a healthy image but many of Müller's products, like its bestselling Corner vanilla yoghurt with chocolate balls, are relatively high in sugar (16g/100g). As with CSDs, there are lighter (reduced sugar) versions of many yoghurts, but like fizzy drinks, these contain sweeteners such as Aspartame and Acesulfame K, which have the same potential health issues that were highlighted earlier.

Danone with sales of £295m is number 2 in the highly competitive UK yoghurt market. Its Activia brand makes a big play on gut health, but many of its products also contain added sugar, as do many of the products targeting kids like Yoplait's Petit Filous. As public health authorities waged war on saturated fat, the yoghurt producers adapted their offer so that many products carry a low-fat claim. The flip side, as I pointed out already, is that low fat often means high sugar. As the science and understanding behind saturated fats is evolving, you can once again find more and more full fat dairy yoghurts.

My personal preference is for full fat Greek yoghurt, which has all the texture and creaminess you could wish for but is relatively low in sugar and has a correspondingly low glycaemic index (GI). As with many other food categories, the simpler and more natural the product, the better it is for you. But beware poor alternatives. To make true Greek yoghurt requires 100kg of milk for every 40kg of yoghurt. My brand of choice is Fage Total 5% which is made the traditional 'strained' way. Other brands prefer to take shortcuts and use the descriptor 'Greek-style' that betrays the fact that it is a poor imitation, often with additives to try and create the same texture and creaminess as the real thing.

Trolley recommendation:

Full-fat natural yoghurt (e.g. Fage Total

5%)
Sweetened low-fat yoghurt

Fruit juices/fruit smoothies

Before we look at this category in more detail let's delve a little deeper into the Glycaemic Index (GI) and why it matters. Here is a good definition from the Harvard Medical Journal (first published in 2015):

"The glycaemic index is a value assigned to foods based on how slowly or how quickly those foods cause increases in blood glucose levels. Foods low on the glycaemic index (GI) scale tend to release glucose slowly and steadily. Foods high on the glycaemic index release glucose rapidly. Low GI foods tend to foster weight loss, while foods high on the GI scale help with energy recovery after exercise, or to offset hypo- (or insufficient) glycaemia. Long-distance runners would tend to favour foods high on the glycaemic index, while people with pre- or full-blown diabetes would need to concentrate on low GI foods. Why? People with type 1 diabetes cannot produce sufficient quantities of insulin and those with type 2 diabetes are resistant to insulin. With both types of diabetes, faster glucose release from high GI foods leads to spikes in blood sugar levels. The slow and steady release of glucose in low-glycaemic foods helps maintain good glucose control."

So, unless you are a marathon runner, GI is something you need to be paying attention to in order to keep your blood glucose levels under control.

Tropicana, owned by PepsiCo, is the leading fruit juice brand in the UK with sales of £212m. PepsiCo's big rival Coca Cola owns the market-leading fruit smoothies brand, Innocent, which, with sales of £264m, is the UK's 24th biggest grocery brand. PepsiCo and Coca Cola know all about selling sugar and water through their CSD brands. Fructose, the principal sugar in fruit juices, is just sugar in another form. Over the last few years, the government has been educating us about the importance of eating '5-a-day', i.e. 5 portions of fruit and vegetables a day. How you get your 5-a-day is probably more important than the what.

Here is what Diabetes UK has to say about fruit juices and fruit smoothies versus eating unadulterated whole fruit:

"Fructose adds to your intake of free (added) sugars. Whole fruit, on the other hand, does not. Whole fruit contains fibre (roughage), vitamins and minerals, which are good for your overall health. The fibre helps to slow down the speed the fructose is absorbed into your blood stream and can help you feel fuller for longer. This is why it's better to eat whole fruit, rather than fruit in the form of juice or a smoothie. Fruit juice and smoothies, on the other hand, have most of the fibre (roughage) removed when they are made and it's very easy to drink large quantities in a short space of time. This means you could be drinking a lot of extra calories, carbs and sugar."

Orange juice, e.g. Tropicana, has a GI of between 66 and 76 on a scale of 100, which makes it a very high GI drink. It is not advisable for diabetics but, even if you are not diabetic, too many high GI foods can negatively affect insulin sensitivity, cholesterol levels and blood pressure.

Yet again we are seeing that processing of foods has potentially negative consequences for health. I am not saying never have fruit juice or smoothies but rather that they should be an occasional treat. If you are a regular fruit eater, then eat it whole.

Trolley recommendation:

Tropicana or other natural fruit juice

Biscuits & Cakes

McVitie's, now owned by Turkish giant Pladis, is the UK's 11th biggest grocery brand with sales of over £460m and an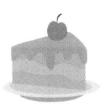

impressive array of brands in its portfolio: HobNobs, Jaffa Cakes, Chocolate Digestives, Rich Tea, Penguin, Club. Who doesn't love a biscuit with their cup of tea? Mr. Kipling, with sales of £167m is the big seller in cakes.

By all means indulge in the occasional biscuit or cake. My issue with industrially produced sweet treats is the amount of additives compared to home baking. It's a given that these products are high sugar (Jaffa Cakes are over 52g of sugar per 100g, making them one of the sweetest treats you can buy). What is less transparent are the E numbers and added chemicals which ensure a long shelf life, stable texture and taste.

For example, Mr Kipling's Unicorn Slices has the following ingredients list:

Sugar, Vegetable Oils (Rapeseed, Palm), Wheat Flour (with Added Calcium, Iron, Niacin, Thiamin), Water, Glucose Syrup, Humectant (Vegetable Glycerine), Dextrose, Dried Egg White, Whey Powder (Milk), Maize Starch, Vegetable Fat (Palm), Raising Agents (Disodium Diphosphate,

Sodium Bicarbonate), Emulsifiers (Mono- and Diglycerides of Fatty Acids, Sorbitan Monostearate, Polyglycerol Esters of Fatty Acids, Soya Lecithin, Polysorbate 60), Skimmed Milk Powder, Tapioca Starch, Salt, Stabiliser (Xanthan Gum), Preservative (Potassium Sorbate), Milk Proteins, Red Beet, Flavourings, Gelling Agent (Sodium Alginate), Colours (Titanium Dioxide, Carmine, Lutein), Acid (Acetic Acid), Spirulina

I wouldn't claim to be an expert on baking cakes, but I bet Mary Berry doesn't use many of the above in her recipes. Once the ingredient list gets beyond half a dozen items, many of which you cannot even pronounce, let alone know what they do, then it's probably a good idea to avoid. Mr Kipling may make exceedingly good cakes, to quote the old advertising, but he does it in a large-scale factory with industrial chemicals and processes.

Ironically, as a nation we love watching TV programmes like The Great British Bake Off, but it has become a spectator sport rather than something we actually do unless we have to. As I write this, the whole country is in lockdown as a result of the Covid-19 pandemic. There are reports that the supermarkets have run out of flour as people are once again turning to home baking. Nigella Lawson, who was arguably well ahead of her time when it comes to home cooking, argues eloquently about the benefits during times like the Coronavirus crisis:

"Touching things, smelling something, listening. Baking really has so much of that, because when you're kneading dough or you're stirring a bowl, you are really immersed in the world of the senses. And that's really very important, because otherwise you're trapped in your mind, and that isn't now a very comfortable place."

So, there you have it. Baking is so much more than producing something nice to eat, it can also be very therapeutic! Less factory food and more homemade cakes and we will all be better off in more ways than you think.

Trolley recommendation:

Branded cakes & biscuits
Flour & other home baking
ingredients

Frozen Food (Savoury)

Birds Eye with sales of nearly £490m, McCain (£320m) and Young's Seafood (£180m) are the leading frozen food brands in the UK. I am a big fan of frozen food, not least because of the increasing issue of food waste. Frozen food is convenient, value for money, usually minimally packaged and generally means less waste. 98% of UK households own a freezer and we consume around 29kg of frozen food per head every year. This is still only around 5% by value of our total grocery shopping. The big frozen categories (excluding ice-cream) are fish, potato products, pizza, ready meals, meat & poultry, and vegetables.

I will talk about ready meals in more detail later in the context of chilled food. When buying frozen food, the same basic principles apply as in other categories: the less processed (the shorter the ingredient list) the better. Frozen vegetables in their unadulterated, natural form, e.g. peas, beans, broccoli, are a good staple to have in your freezer. The big frozen food brands prefer to sell their 'added value' products that have been processed, to a greater or lesser extent, on their factory production lines. Generally speaking, the more processed, the higher the profit margin. So, Birds Eye's bestselling potato waffles contain a lot more than just potato: Potato (88%), Rapeseed Oil, Potato Granules, Potato Starch, Salt, Stabiliser (Hydroxypropyl Methylcellulose), White Pepper.

Similarly, McCain's top selling French Fries have an industrial batter and are fried in sunflower oil. Big Food loves to market sunflower oil as healthy but it's not so straightforward. There is evidence that certain types of sunflower oil are toxic when heated above 82 degrees Celsius, e.g. during frying potatoes [1]. When I was young, a Friday night chip shop supper was a frequent treat. Back in those days, beef dripping was the fat used by most chip shops, and also most households with a deep fat frying pan. Those were the days before saturated fats like dripping started getting a bad press, and over the years we have been encouraged to replace animal fats with 'healthy' polyunsaturated vegetable oils. In home cooking, oil is normally used only once or twice before being thrown away. In food factories that run 24-7, oil is used and abused over and over again for up to two weeks. Industrial specification oils are known as RBD: refined, bleached, and deodorised so that they can stand the rigours of factory processing over several days of intensive use. Manufacturers will also often add chemical 'improving agents' to maximise longevity and extend the 'fry-life' of the oils they use. You won't see any of these agents on the ingredients list, as they count as 'processing aids' not additives.

Many of the big brand best sellers are deep fried products. Birds Eye Chicken Dippers is apparently made from 100% chicken breast but if you check the ingredients list only contains 50% chicken plus a range of vegetable oils. Birds Eye cod fish fingers are similarly only 58% cod and fried in rapeseed oil. Youngs Chip Shop Large Cod fillets are only 54% fish and list rapeseed oil, sunflower oil, and palm oil in their ingredients. Here is a radical suggestion: buy some cod (100% fish) and fry it at home. It works out cheaper and it is better for you.

Aunt Bessie's is another of the big, branded players in frozen and was recently acquired by Birds Eye from Hull-based William Jackson Foods. Their potato products and Yorkshire Puddings contain many of the same additives as McCain but overall, the ingredients list is relatively short and on an occasional basis wouldn't kill you.

Frozen pizza is a huge category in its own right with two brands - Chicago Town (Sales £125m) and Dr Oetker (£96m) in the top 100. Pizza Express is sandwiched between the two at number 84 with sales of £107m but is technically a chilled product. Chicago Town's bestselling Deep Dish Pepperoni Pizza contains a host of nasty additives, including preservatives, sugar, starches, E-numbers, and artificial flavourings. If you are going to treat yourself to a pizza then probably best to buy a chilled one (with fewer additives) or, even better, buy some dough (or make your own dough from scratch) and add your own toppings. It is really pretty easy and works out a lot cheaper.

Trolley recommendation:

Peas & frozen vegetables
Frozen fish (natural)
Oven chips/potato products
Battered & breaded meat & fish
Frozen pizza

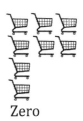

Zero

Ice Cream

One of the features of the food industry is the on-going product innovation that creates new brands and categories. Much of this innovation comes from smaller start-ups who identify a gap in the market where they can enter without being squashed by

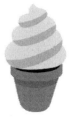

the 900lb gorillas prowling the food jungle and defending their territory. Examples include brands like Fever Tree in the drinks market, Innocent Smoothies and Tyrrells potato crisps. One of my favourite business gurus, Brian Tracy, loves to say, 'there's always room at the top', meaning that premium, high quality products and services will always find willing buyers. It is no surprise that many of the successful food innovations of recent years tend to be premium offerings – and nowhere more so than the ice cream market.

One of the reasons that a gap often appears at the top is that Big Food over time tends to remove quality from its products by 'reengineering' recipes and introducing cheaper ingredients to improve profit margins. The first major super-premium ice-cream brand was Haagen-Dazs, founded in 1961 in New York by Reuben Mattus, who invented the brand name because it sounded Danish. He had a soft spot for Denmark and associated the country with quality dairy products. The original Haagen-Dazs recipe was very dense (with little air mixed in during manufacture), had a high cream and butterfat content and used no emulsifiers or stabilisers (other than egg yolks). Today the brand in the UK is owned by North American MNC General Mills and it remains one of the most indulgent ice creams on the market with 31% fresh cream, although it does now use emulsifiers and gelling agents in its recipe.

The biggest ice cream brand in the UK is Unilever owned Magnum, which is worth nearly £200m at retail. This is the ingredients list for a Magnum Classic (vanilla ice cream with chocolate):

Reconstituted skimmed milk, sugar, cocoa butter, whey concentrate (milk), cocoa mass, coconut oil, glucose syrup, glucose-fructose syrup, whole milk powder, butter oil, emulsifiers (E471, SOYA lecithin, E476), stabilisers (E410, E412, E407), vanilla bean pieces, flavourings, colour (E160a).

There are more Es in that list than you'll find on a Scrabble board and the number one ingredient is not even cream. So, by any definition Magnum is not even close to being the best ice cream on the market, but it is by far and away the best seller. This is testament to the marketing muscle and distribution power of its owner Unilever, one of the biggest food producers on the planet.

The Anglo-Dutch manufacturer also owns the number two ice cream brand on the UK market, Ben & Jerry's. Ben Cohen and Jerry Greenfield were childhood friends in New York who learned how to make ice cream before opening their first ice cream parlour in Vermont in 1979. They quickly grew to challenge Haagen-Dazs's leadership of the premium sector and the two founders also gained a reputation for championing social causes, e.g. animal welfare and children's charities. The book of their journey focuses on "How Two Real Guys Built a Business with a Social Conscience and a Sense of Humour" and is a real-life example of how start-ups with a quality product and innovative marketing can compete with Big Food. In 2000, however, Ben and Jerry sold to Unilever and a lot of the magic went out of the business. With the main ice cream brands once again belonging to faceless MNCs, I am predicting that it won't be long before another innovative challenger pops up with something better in this category.

Clearly the obesity crisis in the UK is not going to be solved by eating ice cream but there must be room in life for a little treat every now and again. Personally, if I eat ice cream then I want a product where the number one ingredient is cream, and I don't need a magnifying glass to read all the ingredients. There are still a few brands out there that meet these criteria, but you have to look beyond the current market leader.

Trolley recommendation:

Haagen-Dazs or other high cream brand

Cook-in Sauces

In April 2016 Mars Food, the owner of Dolmio and Uncle Ben's, advised customers that some of its products were so high in sugar, fat and salt that

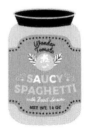

they shouldn't be eaten more than once a week. Yes, you read that correctly, a food company advised its customers to buy less of its own product. I should disclose something at this point. I spent over a decade of my career working at Mars and have something of a soft spot for them. Unusually for a large MNC they are still family-owned and although no longer running the business, the Mars siblings still have a big say in how the company is run. Their private ownership has always allowed Mars to take a longer-term, more ethical view of business than some of its publicly listed competitors who are more concerned with today's share price and cannot see beyond the next set of quarterly results. It is hard to imagine the executives at Kraft-Heinz or Coca-Cola altruistically advising consumers to restrict consumption. Corporate America will do virtually anything to maintain sales and profits and drive their share price higher. They will push the boundaries of what is legal or ethical and then use highly paid lawyers to defend their position. That is what makes Mars' announcement so unusual.

Despite the health warnings, Dolmio still has sales of over £100m and ranks in the Top 100 UK grocery brands. Even after working there I am still a little baffled about the success of Dolmio. Take their standard 500g original Bolognese sauce, which has the following ingredients and retails for about £1.85:

Tomatoes (78%), Tomato Paste (10%), Onion, Sugar, Modified Maize Starch, Salt, Sunflower Oil, Basil (0.3%), Garlic, Acidity Regulator (Citric Acid), Parsley, Herb, Spices

Now I am no Jamie Oliver but even I can knock together a tomato sauce. Here is my ingredients list:

Chopped tomatoes (tinned or fresh), tablespoon of tomato paste (puree), chopped onion, crushed clove of garlic, olive oil, mixed Italian herbs, salt & pepper.

My recipe does not contain any added sugar, modified starch or acidity regulators. It is dead easy to make (about 15 minutes) and costs a fraction of a jar of Dolmio. I know I am biased, but I think it tastes better and doesn't leave that unpleasant after-taste of mass-produced factory food. The same principles apply to other cook-in sauces like curry. The number one ingredient in Patak's Tikka Masala sauce is water! If you have been paying attention, then you'll recall that water is virtually free in this country. All you need to do is invest in a spice rack and you can make most standard sauces with very little difficulty, at a fraction of the cost and with none of the nasty additives. Give it a go and I promise you, you will never buy a branded sauce ever again.

Trolley recommendation:

Take Mars' advice!

Cheese

We Brits like a bit of cheese with each of us consuming on average about 30g/day. This

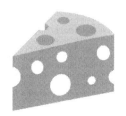

may sound like a lot, but it is only half of the level of the French and Italians. We are also not particularly adventurous with over half of our total cheese consumption being one variety: cheddar. Personally, I don't mind a bit of cheddar but it's a bit like buying your underwear in M&S: safe but not very exciting. Surprisingly, there are over 700 varieties of cheese produced in the UK, so it's not like we don't have enough choice. Our predilection for cheddar lies behind the remarkable success of Cathedral City. With sales of over £270m it is the 25th biggest brand in the UK. It is decent cheddar made in Cornwall and comes in a convenient re-sealable pack but is it really worth paying over the odds for? It is roughly twice the price per kilo of retailer own-label mature cheddar and once again highlights the important role of marketing in food, even in a commoditised category like cheese.

From a nutrition and health standpoint my preference is for unpasteurised cheese. Brands like Activia and Yakult have successfully exploited the trend for 'gut health' through probiotics but there are more natural (sugar-free!) ways to manage the bacteria in your system. Fermented foods, like cheese, are a potentially rich source of probiotics. The pasteurisation process, however, effectively destroys all the life-giving bacteria. Unpasteurised products do admittedly carry a risk of EHEC (an unpleasant, toxin producing gastroenteritis bacteria) but this is a result of poor hygiene and animal husbandry on some farms and is not a given. Unpasteurised cheeses can still be found on the deli counter in some of our supermarkets (usually imported from France) and are one of the few remaining natural food sources of probiotic gut bacteria.

The other big 'cheese' brand in our supermarket aisles is Dairylea with sales of £127m. I use the term 'cheese' loosely with Dairylea as this industrial version bears only a passing resemblance to traditionally produced cheese. The following description of how processed cheese is made was taken from a well-known food website (foodcrumbles.com):

"Where regular cheese making starts with milk, processed cheese production actually starts with cheese! The manufacturer will choose one or several cheeses they want to include in the processed cheese. These cheeses are then grated and melted. The melted cheese is mixed with other ingredients again. Common additional ingredients are (which are allowed depends on the country the cheese is made and sold):

- Milk fats
- Other dairy ingredients: whey proteins are quite common
- Emulsifying salts: these modify the proteins in the cheese such that they are dispersed better which makes for this very homogeneous product.
- Salt (processed cheese tends to contain more salt than regular cheese)
- Colourings and spices

The ingredients are heated and mixed to make a stable mass. Heating is required to pasteurise the product. Both the way the processed cheese is processed as well as the ingredients strongly influence the final properties. It has been found that the cook time, cook temperature, extent of

101

mixing as well as rate of cooling all influence the final processed cheese properties."

Doesn't exactly sound appetising does it? Kraft's marketing team in the USA once christened processed cheese 'liquid gold' and they have successfully developed a range of kid's products around it with the somewhat spurious health claim that they are "a good source of calcium". This is rather like claiming that chocolate is a good source of milk. A few years ago, Dairylea's boast that their Lunchables were "full of good stuff" was banned by the UK's Advertising Standards Authority (ASA) largely because of the high levels of fat and salt in the product. Their best-selling Dunkers product retails at a pricey £2.25 for some 'liquid gold' and a few crisps. (I would list the ingredients but with all the additives it would probably double the word count of this book.) This works out at nearly £12/kilo, which is more than double the price of real mature cheddar. But hey, it is a 'good source of calcium'! As you can probably tell I am not a big fan of Dairylea. Their owners Kraft-Heinz have a dubious track record in marketing unhealthy products to children and I see very little in the Dairylea range to commend it. Still it sells in lorry loads thanks in part to the marketing machine behind the brand, which exports best practice to the UK from the United States, which is, lest we forget, the most obese major country in the world.

Trolley recommendation:

Quality unpasteurised cheese
Other real cheese (e.g. cheddar)
Processed cheese

Zero

Savoury Snacks

Back in 1986 I was a student in Germany and ran around punching the air of my apartment when Gary Lineker ignited England's World Cup campaign with a hat trick against Poland on his way to winning the coveted Golden Boot. I went on to a career in the Food industry while Lineker has become a successful TV presenter and also the front man for Walkers crisps, the UK's biggest savoury snack brand worth nearly £1 billion. Ironically, it was the future Chairman of the Football Association, Martin Glenn, who, as a PepsiCo marketer, had the brainwave to recruit Lineker to front the marketing push behind Walkers in 1995. The business was originally founded in Leicester in 1948 and was acquired by Frito-Lay, a division of US MNC PepsiCo, in 1989. Typically, when US brands acquire local independent companies, they quickly ditch the local brand and adopt their own global branding. So, for example, wherever Frito-Lay operates they use the Lays brand for potato crisps (or potato chips as they call them in America). Walkers has been such an outstanding success, however, and has such a dominant market leadership position (5 times the size of its nearest competitor), that Frito-Lay have retained the Walkers brand and kept faith with Lineker in the longest running major marketing campaign ever seen in the UK.

We Brits love a bag of crisps, consuming around 6 billion packets a year (that is a staggering 150 packets each). If it's not a bag of Walkers then you'll likely find us munching on one of the other big brands: Pringles (now owned by Kellogg's), Doritos (a stable mate of Walkers under Frito-Lay), Hula Hoops or McCoy's (both part of KP Snacks). These brands, together with Walkers, generate over £1.6bn of annual sales. Add in brands like Tyrrells, Kettle Chips and all the retail own-label offerings and you have one of the biggest and most profitable categories in UK grocery. In many ways, potato crisps are the holy grail of processed food: a cheap and plentiful raw material that can be relatively easily transformed into a delicious, moreish product that can be sold at a huge profit.

In chapter 1 I talked about the dangers of acrylamide in crisps and other fried products. Crisps also tend to be very high in calories (e.g. a third of a pack of Pringles contains over 300 calories), high in fat and salt. Given the excessive consumption of crisps this is one area where UK consumers could theoretically easily cut down. PepsiCo (Frito-Lay), Kellogg's, KP Snacks and others have driven consumption of unhealthy salty snacks to staggeringly high levels, which are inarguably having negative health consequences for British consumers. Is it not misleading and disingenuous for a slim, fit-looking ex-professional footballer to extol the supposed virtues of eating crisps? I spent several years coaching junior football and the boys were encouraged to bring a drink and snack to training to refuel at the end of the session. I was shocked at how many of them brought along a bag of crisps (and often a bar of chocolate). At the time McDonalds was the Football Association's main sponsor (replaced later by Mars Bars) and Lineker, as he still does today, was presenting Match of The Day. It is outrageous that junk food should be favourably associated with physical activity, especially children's sport. But despite the ASA's efforts, Big Food still looks to corrupt and create new addicts wherever possible. An occasional packet (say one per week) is acceptable but consumption at the rate we see in the UK is a national scandal.

If you do want to eat a regular savoury snack, then ditch the crisps and start eating nuts. Nuts are high in fat, low in carbs, and a great source of several nutrients, including vitamin E, magnesium, and selenium. They have also been shown to lower the risk of diabetes and heart disease. Try to eat nuts in their unprocessed, natural state, i.e. without any added oil or salt. A handful a day is all you need to potentially add to your life expectancy [2].

Trolley recommendation:

Crisps & processed potato snacks (Walkers or another brand)
Unprocessed nuts & seeds

Confectionery

The list of the UK's top grocery brands is chock full of some of our favourite sweet treats: Cadbury, Nestlé, Lindt, 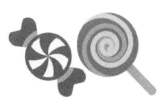 Galaxy, Maltesers, Kinder, Haribo, Rowntree's, Maynards Bassetts, M&Ms, Mars, Ferrero. No other food category comes close to having so many brands in the top 100. Cadbury sales alone are worth a staggering £1.7billion, making it the biggest single brand on our shelves.

Chocolate confectionery is a category I know well from my time at Mars and our love of chocolate goes back a long way. When Forrest Mars Senior arrived in England on the boat from America in the 1930s, all he had was a few dollars and a recipe for a chocolate bar, to which we would give his name. Forrest started hand making Mars bars in a rudimentary shed in Slough, on the site where now sits one of the biggest chocolate factories in the world. Roald Dahl used the factory as his inspiration for Willy Wonka and today it continues to churn out Mars bars alongside Snickers, Bounty, Maltesers, Galaxy and other household names. Together with Cadbury and Rowntree's of York (now part of Nestlé), Mars for many years was part of a triumvirate that shaped the UK chocolate market and turned it into one of the most profitable food categories in the world. These three companies made chocolate affordable and accessible for the masses. A product that had previously been an occasional luxury treat became an everyday purchase. In the case of the Mars bar this was for many years literally the message behind the brand: A Mars a Day Helps You Work Rest and Play. Well, until you get Type 2 diabetes that is.

In recent years, traditional big-selling bars like Mars and Snickers have seen a decline. This has been partly self-inflicted. As we mentioned earlier (see cook-in sauces section) Mars Inc. (the company) is unusual in having a greater sense of social responsibility than most. A few years ago, they took the proactive decision to reduce the size of their products to cut calories in recognition of the growing obesity crisis in the UK. A Snickers bar now weighs 48g, a Mars bar only 51g (down from a peak of 65g) and both products contain fewer than 250 calories. As altruistic a move as this was, it has undoubtedly reduced the value for money and affected sales. This has been compounded by a shift in consumer tastes towards higher quality block chocolate. Swiss confectioner Lindt has seen significant growth in recent years with their premium, higher cocoa-based products. Mars has helped offset declining sales of its traditional bars with growth of the indulgent Galaxy brand. Chocolate can be one of life's great pleasures but for too many people it has become an everyday staple, consumed in far too great a quantity. The chocolate makers are fully aware of this and even secretly nurture their brand's 'heavy users'. Such customers eat more than a bar a day and often several. They are a huge source of sales and profit and later in life you will often find them being wheeled into hospital with diet and weight related conditions.

The food industry has long resisted comparisons with tobacco, claiming that what they sell is not addictive. I beg to differ. There is compelling evidence that sugar is addictive. One chocolate bar never killed anybody just like one cigarette never killed anybody. If we all ate only one chocolate bar a week then there would be much less obesity and the big chocolate producers would have much smaller businesses. Big Food is greedier than its consumers. It has created an addiction to sugar to fuel its own addiction to profits. I am not saying totally give up on chocolate. Personally, I love a bit of Lindt 70% Cocoa. But if you are one of the people eating a bar/day or more then think about cutting down. The advice in this chapter is all interconnected. Eating 3 meals/day of healthy, unprocessed food will significantly reduce the urge to snack on chocolate. Like any addiction it is possible to wean yourself off it.

Trolley Recommendation:

High quality dark chocolate, e.g. Lindt 70%

The other main type of non-chocolate confectionery is sugar. Brands like Haribo, Rowntree's and Maynards Bassetts are the big players in this sub-category, often unashamedly targeting kids (or their parents) with their marketing. Like fruit juice, sugar confectionery has an extremely high GI. A 100g portion of Haribo Starmix is 342 calories, of which nearly half is pure sugar and will give you an insulin spike higher than the bounce back on a bungee rope. Never ones to miss out on a trend lest it damage sales, you can now also find reduced sugar versions of sugar confectionery. This seems to me the equivalent of selling orange juice with slightly fewer oranges in it. 100g of Haribo Fruitilicious 30% Reduced Sugar sweets still contain 282 calories so you might wonder what is the point? Again, I don't want to be a complete killjoy so I'm not saying never eat sugar confectionery – but only use it as a treat not a daily snack. You will see a lot less of your dentist too.

Trolley recommendation:

(Maybe the odd wine gum when you're out walking the dog)

Chilled Ready Meals

You will not find any chilled ready meal brands in the list of Britain's biggest grocery brands. This is a market that the big retailers have largely cornered for themselves so when you wander down the chilled food aisle the products bear the supermarket's own branding. I have decided to cover ready meals in this book because we all eat them from time to time and for many shoppers, they are a frequent purchase. Chilled convenience food is very big business – over £10 billion a year – which represents around 13% of the UK's total retail food market. Over the years a few branded manufacturers have tried to enter this lucrative market but, with the possible exception of Charlie Bigham's, operating at the premium end, few have succeeded.

One of the pioneers of the UK ready meal industry was Gulam Noon, an Indian immigrant, who started manufacturing chilled and frozen Indian and Thai ready meals for UK supermarkets in the late 1980s. His business, Noon Products, grew rapidly, thanks largely to a fruitful partnership with Sainsbury's, and many credit him with the popularity of chicken tikka masala in Britain. Sir Gulam (as he became) boldly asserted that he "changed the palate of the nation, and broke the housewife's shackles from the kitchen." Noon Products was eventually taken over by Irish food giant, Kerry Foods, and today a vast network of chilled food factories exists to serve our growing appetite for convenience products. Many of these companies are large businesses in their own right

- Samworths, Bakkavor, 2 Sisters, Greencore - but you will rarely see their names as the products coming out of their factories invariably carry the retailers' brand.

A chilled food factory is not exactly a fun place to work. There is a healthy obsession with food safety, which means the ambient temperature inside is kept at 2-4 degrees Celsius and there is no natural light. It's akin to working in a fridge with the light on. For many low-paid (often immigrant) workers these inhospitable factories are the modern-day equivalent of going down the coalmines.

But what of the products they churn out? Are they really a godsend to modern day housewives? Are they as good as, or better than homemade? In a word, no. Not by a long way. Food produced on an industrial scale uses processes and ingredients that are a world apart from your kitchen at home. Home cooking inevitably involves variability – no homemade sauce, pie or stew tastes exactly the same every time you make it for a whole host of reasons: differences in ingredients, cooking time, seasonality, different quantities of meat or veg, added salt, etc. Factories are all about standardisation as per this extract from a government food safety manual: 'To achieve a consistent product with the same appearance, flavour, shelf life, etc., it is important that the ingredient quantities, quality and the processing steps are always the same.'

Most chilled ready meals leave the factory with about 28 days shelf life. I challenge you to make a meal at home that will keep for nearly a month in your fridge. Chilled food manufacturers have done a good job in seemingly cleaning up the ingredients list on their products, but most are still worryingly long. Moreover, what you do not see is the cooking process and the addition of colourings and food processing aids to ensure the product can survive a month in the supply chain before consumption. The proof of the pudding is, as always, in the eating, and factory produced ready meals always leave an unpleasant after-taste on the palate that you rarely get with home-cooked food. The size of the chilled ready meals market in the UK (per capita the largest in the world) reflects our increasing prioritisation of convenience over taste. Most ready meals are a poor substitute for scratch cooking in virtually every respect: taste, nutrition and value for money. Sir Gulam may have helped break the housewife's shackles but he did not change our palates for the better.

Trolley recommendation:

Canned Food

For most of their existence humans have lived in times of scarcity. In abundant times, therefore, they developed ways to preserve excess food stocks: drying, smoking, pickling,  fermenting etc. At the turn of the 19th century Napoleon and his armies were marching around Europe picking battles with their neighbours near and far. As Napoleon himself astutely observed, an army marches on its stomach and his particular army needed a lot of food. This led to the French government offering a cash award to any inventor who could devise a cheap and effective method of preserving large amounts of food to fuel French military ambitions. Ultimately this led to the development of the canning process (albeit too late for Napoleon to benefit from) and this was gradually employed in other European countries and in the US.

Canned foods remain highly popular today, providing a shelf life of one to five years in a convenient, practical format. Nutritionally it has been shown that canned foods are, in some instances, better than the fresh or frozen equivalents. For instance, canned tomatoes have a higher available lycopene content than fresh tomatoes. As with many of the previous categories it is best to look for canned food that has not been overly processed (beyond the canning process itself). So tinned tuna, tomatoes, kidney beans and lentils are all great things to have in your cupboard.

The most popular canned food in the UK, however, is that versatile favourite the baked bean – the UK eats more cans of baked beans than the rest of the world combined - and the leading brand is Heinz. A staggering 1.5 million cans of Heinz Beanz are sold every day in the UK.

The Heinz canning factory near Wigan is one of the largest in the world, producing, alongside its iconic beans, soups, macaroni cheese and spaghetti hoops. Heinz products unfortunately tend to have a couple of common denominators: lots of sugar and lots of salt. I am a big fan of pulses like beans (even when canned) but cover them in sickly sweet tomato sauce and you undo a lot of the nutritional benefit. Half a can of beans would give you more than 20% of your recommended daily salt intake.

The longevity of the can is based on its proven performance as a robust, efficient, safe packaging format. Compared to other categories, food manufacturers have tended not to use it to sell junk. But there are still products that should be avoided or at the very least consumed less frequently. Baked beans, spaghetti hoops and soups fall into that category.

Trolley recommendation:

Canned pulses, beans, vegetables, fish, tomatoes
Baked beans, canned soups

Vegetarian/Vegan/Free-from

In the interests of transparency, I should disclose here that I am an unashamed carnivore.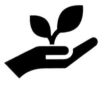
Nonetheless I respect the fact that for many people eating animals is not an option, either for ethical or other reasons. I can't offer any fresh insight here into the arguments for or against vegetarianism or veganism. What I can usefully do is help you better understand the meat-free options that Big Food companies would like you to buy in the supermarket.

Food manufacturers tend to be ambivalent about new consumer trends leading to product innovation. Reformulating recipes, setting up new supplier agreements, getting legal approvals, reconfiguring factories, negotiating new listings with retailers, and producing new advertising all costs time and expensive resources. Moreover, food product innovation has a staggeringly high failure rate - some measures put the chances of success, i.e. still in market three years post launch, at less than 10%. Vegetarianism and veganism appears to be a trend that is becoming increasingly mainstream and Big Food wants a piece of the action. We saw earlier how Upfield, the makers of Flora margarine, are keen to emphasise the plant-based credentials of their products, as if plant-based in itself was a virtue, regardless of the real nutritional content. This is what I would define as pure opportunism, i.e. a highly processed brand, that just happens to be meat-free, jumping on the vegetarian bandwagon.

There are brands, however, which owe their very existence to the need to find alternatives to animal-based food. Let's take a look at the two biggest, starting with dairy-alternative brand Alpro, which is now worth over £220m in sales. Alpro's main products comprise a range of nut 'milks' that are marketed as an alternative to cow's milk for people who are either lactose intolerant or who are seeking a vegan/vegetarian alternative to traditional dairy.

Of course, nut 'milk' is something of a misnomer – nuts don't produce milk, mammals do! Alpro wants you to believe that their products are the plant-based equal of cow's milk. Let's be crystal clear – they're not. Cow's milk is a 100% natural, highly nutritious source of calcium and protein. Nut 'milks' are highly processed with lots of additives. Take the ingredients list for Alrpo's unsweetened almond 'milk':

Water, Almond (2.3%), Calcium (Tri-Calcium Phosphate), Sea Salt, Stabilisers (Locust Bean Gum, Gellan Gum), Emulsifier (Lecithins (Sunflower)), Vitamins (B2, B12, E, D2)

Even with all the additives, almond 'milk' still only contains a fraction of the protein of cow's milk and is not suitable to give to infants under 3 years old. Alpro's bestselling soya 'milk' is admittedly higher in protein than almond 'milk' but still contains all the above additives. Soy has, however, been linked with breast cancer and the NHS advises anyone who has been diagnosed with this type of cancer to avoid soy products [3].

Many people look to dairy alternatives because they suffer from allergies or intolerances to the proteins found in cow's milk. If you are not lactose intolerant then there is little justification on health or nutrition grounds to consume nut 'milks' instead of cow's milk. You will also be better off financially. Nut 'milks' are roughly twice the cost of real milk.

The other brand successfully riding the new wave of popularity for meat-free eating is the meat analogue brand Quorn, which is now the 39th biggest brand in the UK, worth an impressive £188m. The brand owes its existence to a joint venture between food company Rank Hovis McDougall (RHM) and Imperial Chemical Industries (ICI) dating back to the 1980s. ICI actually started the research in the 1960s with the intention of finding a food that could be produced in a windowless nuclear bunker in the event of Armageddon. All Quorn products contain mycoprotein as the main ingredient, which is derived from the *Fusarium venenatum* fungus. In most cases the fungus culture is dried and mixed with egg albumen, which acts as a binder, and then is adjusted in texture and pressed into various forms. A vegan formulation also exists that uses potato protein as a binder instead of egg albumen.

Here's the ingredient list for Quorn 'Chicken Style Fillets':

Mycoprotein™ (85%), Rehydrated Free-Range Egg White, Natural Flavouring, Firming Agents: Calcium Chloride, Calcium Acetate, Gelling Agent: Pectin

What baffles me slightly about overtly virtue-signalling vegetarian brands is how much they want you to think they are like meat. Quorn has borrowed unashamedly from meat marketing - burgers, sausages, bacon, peppered steaks, crunchy nuggets – are all part of the extensive range of products. Remember what you are

123

actually eating is largely 'mycoprotein' – don't be fooled by the trademark, it's a fungus grown in a laboratory, mixed with chemicals and processing aids to give it the texture of meat. I think I'll stick with a free-range chicken breast or a grass-fed fillet steak. I know that is not an option for vegetarians but even if I did give up meat, I'd like to think I could do better than Quorn.

Just in case you think I am picking on Quorn, it's the same story with other brands. The Linda McCartney (LM) brand was one of the first mass market meat-free brands. The packaging proudly bears this statement from her family:

"Mum believed that the kitchen was the heart of the home and we are proud to carry on her ethos of honest, delicious vegetarian food that's good for animals, the earth and you."

I am sorry Linda, but this is just disingenuous claptrap. A pack of LM sausages is full of undesirable ingredients like rehydrated textured soya protein, sulphites, rapeseed oil, ammonium bicarbonate and methyl cellulose, to name just a few. I struggle to believe that Mrs. Macca had any of these ingredients in her kitchen cupboard. It is just more processed junk masquerading as healthy behind a vegetarian banner. 'Plant-based' and 'Plant power' have become the new buzzwords for food companies looking to exploit the growing demand for vegetarian and vegan products. You need to look behind the slogans and use your own judgement as to whether the products are as virtuous and healthy as the manufacturers would have you believe. The same applies to other free-from categories like gluten free. The leading gluten free bread brand, Promise, is still essentially a Chorleywood-style loaf with a lengthy ingredients list of thickeners, preservatives, and other chemicals. It might stop you getting ill from gluten but what else is it doing to your body?

Trolley recommendation:

Real vegetables (in their natural, unprocessed state)
Meat substitutes   Zero

Organic

If you went shopping at Tesco back in 2016 you could by 'butcher's quality cuts' meat from Boswell 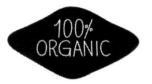 Farms, succulent cherry tomatoes from Nightingale Farms, baby carrots from Redmere Farms and chicken mini fillets from Willow Farms. You can buy produce from these typically English sounding places, but you can't locate them on a map. They don't exist. They are fake – the invention of Tesco marketing department. Dave Lewis, Tesco's CEO, credited the fake farms with an uplift in sales of fresh produce at his stores. He showed little remorse when challenged on the ethics of such marketing. Tesco is not alone in using this ploy. Many of the other retailers also 'invent' farms to give their produce a better image, although Morrisons have now said they will no longer do this.

Does it matter? Is it any different to Premier Foods pretending the avuncular Mr Kipling makes their cakes? In my view it is another example of how the large corporations, in this case the big retailers, are deliberately misleading shoppers and creating opacity where there should be transparency. Consumers have a right to know where their food comes from. Farming is of huge strategic, environmental, economic, and cultural importance. It is also at the heart of understanding the debate around organic food.

Other than Yeo Valley (with sales of over £150m) there are no 100% organic brands in the list of the UK's top 100 grocery brands although some of the big boys do offer organic versions of their products, e.g. Heinz ketchup and baked beans. Organic food has been available in our supermarkets for a long time but has not yet become mainstream. I believe that a large part of the reason for this is lack of clarity about the benefits of buying organic. To help demystify this category let's look at some definitions with the help of the Soil Association, the charitable body responsible for the certification of organic food in the UK.

The Soil Association describes organic food as follows:

'All organic food is fully traceable from farm to fork, so you can be sure of what you're eating. The standards for organic food are laid down in European law so any food labelled as organic must meet strict rules. Unlike non-organic food production, which makes wide use of manufactured and mined fertilisers and pesticides, organic food is produced with natural fertilisers from plants, less energy and more respect for the animals that provide it. Organic farming and food production is not easy and takes real commitment and attention to detail, and is backed up by rigorous, independent inspection and certification.'

So that is the 'what' - but why should you buy organic food? Again, the Soil Association explains:

'Organic means working with nature. It means higher levels of animal welfare, lower levels of pesticides, no manufactured herbicides or artificial fertilisers and more environmentally sustainable management of the land and natural environment, which means more wildlife.

Whatever you are buying – from cotton buds to carrots – when you choose organic food, drink or beauty and textiles, you choose products that promote a better world. Organic food comes from trusted sources. All organic farms and food companies are inspected at least once a year and the standards for organic food are laid down in European law.'

To expand on this, there are several key arguments for organic food over non-organic (the following are again taken from the Soil Association website):

1. Fewer pesticides: Almost 300 pesticides can be routinely used in non-organic farming and are often present in non-organic food.
2. No artificial colours and preservatives: Hydrogenated fats and controversial artificial food colours and preservatives are banned under organic standards.

3. Always free range: Organic means the very highest standards of animal welfare & animals reared without the routine use of drugs, antibiotics & wormers.

4. No routine use of antibiotics: In organic farming systems, animals are reared without the routine use of drugs, antibiotics and wormers common in intensive livestock farming.

5. Better for wildlife: Organic farms are havens for wildlife and provide homes for bees, birds and butterflies – there is up to 50% more wildlife on organic farms.

6. Better for the planet: No system of farming does more to reduce greenhouse gas emissions from agriculture and protect natural resources.

7. It's nutritionally different: Research published in the British Journal of Nutrition found significant differences between organic and non-organic farming. (See below)

8. No GM ingredients: +1 million tonnes of GM crops are imported each year to feed

non-organic livestock. Organic animals can't be fed on GM feed.

So, there are many good environmental and animal welfare reasons for buying organic, but what about the nutritional content? Below is a summary of the key findings from research carried out in 2014 by a team from Newcastle University and published in the British Journal of Nutrition:

- organic milk and meat contain around 50% more omega-3 fatty acids than non-organic
- organic meat had slightly lower concentrations of two saturated fats
- organic milk and dairy contain slightly higher concentrations of iron, Vitamin E and some carotenoids
- organically produced crops (cereals, fruit and vegetables) contain up to 68% more antioxidants than non-organic.
- organic fruit and veg contain lower concentrations of pesticides and the toxic heavy metal cadmium.

It is clear therefore, that the arguments for organic go well beyond helping the environment and better animal welfare. Organic food is also more nutritious. So why don't we buy more of it? I am guessing you're ahead of me on the answer to this – organic almost invariably comes at a price-premium to non-organic. For many on a budget this premium is too much to pay, which is why organic consumption remains heavily skewed towards the better off in our society.

The most high-profile advocate of organic farming and food is the Prince of Wales who launched the Duchy Originals brand in 1990 as a way of bringing to marketing the food grown on his estate. The top end supermarket chain, Waitrose, effectively took over the management of Duchy Originals in 2010 and there are now 230 products in the range. Organic remains, however, a niche segment in our supermarkets, albeit once again a growing one.

I have relatives who are wheat farmers in Canada and I once visited their farm and asked them about organic. They scoffed and said that the yields would be so poor that they could not justify it. Whether all farming should and could be organic is outside the scope of this book. There are legitimate concerns about the environmental impact of intensive farming methods on both crops and animal, not to mention the debate around GMOs and animal cloning. The main counter argument is the need to feed 7 billion people on the planet in an affordable, sustainable way.

In terms of your weekly shop, if you can afford it, I would recommend switching to organic dairy and, if you do eat meat, organic beef, as a minimum. Certain fruit and vegetables, e.g. kale, spinach, strawberries, apples, and peppers, have been shown to contain higher levels of pesticides, so switching to organic may be wise for these items too. My sense is that, as climate change and caring for our environment, increasingly becomes our number one global priority, the support for organic farming and produce will start to swell. For the time being organic food will remain niche but, whilst it is not yet a major factor in the current obesity debate, will increasingly gain relevance.

Another initiative that is worthy of mention is the Red Tractor logo, which confirms that food and drink has been tracked from farm to basket by independent assessors.

This how the people behind the logo describe their work:

'We are the UK's largest food standards scheme, covering all the areas you care about – animal welfare, food safety, traceability and environmental protection. Working with experts in their fields, we are dedicated to ensuring that families across Britain have access to safe, quality food that has been grown and reared in the UK to our rigorous farming standards. Our team of independent assessors perform checks at every step of the food journey from farm to packet, so that people can be sure that it is traceable, safe and farmed with care.

As the recognised scheme of note with over 46,000 British farmer members, our products contribute over £14 billion to the UK economy and Red Tractor membership provides a route to market to some of the UK's largest customers.

Since our establishment in 2000, our Standards have continually evolved to improve food safety, animal welfare and environmental protection, such that they are now among the best in the world.'

So, if you cannot afford organic, at least try and seek out meat, fruit and vegetables bearing the Red Tractor.

Trolley recommendation:

Yeo Valley or another organic milk & dairy

Organic meat

Red Tractor produce

Chapter 5: Dieting & Weight Management

"I have a great diet. You're allowed to eat anything you want, but you must eat it with naked fat people." Ed Bluestone

If you are someone who never diets or has no desire to manage your weight (either up or down) then you can skip ahead to the next chapter. I should begin by stressing that I am not a medical doctor nor am I a qualified nutritionist. I do, however, have extensive knowledge of food and also decades of reading, studying and experimenting with various weight management strategies. I will share with you what has worked for me and give you some recommended reading so that you can make up your own mind after reading some of the experts in this subject.

I am now in my mid-fifties and at 178cm tall (5ft 11") weighing 70kg (just over 11st) am comfortably within the safe BMI as prescribed by the NHS. Apart from a brief period living in

France, when I developed a fondness for the local wine and soft cheese, this has always been the case. I still love good food, fine wine and real ale so in order to keep my BMI in the safe range I have developed a number of successful strategies based on advice from leading expert dieticians and nutritionists. I recognise that my experience is totally subjective but the more I learn the more I see the thinking on this topic begin to converge. This is the thinking I would like to share with you here.

The first time I seriously engaged with dieting was in 2004, aged 40, on my return from France. A couple of years of daily baguettes, cheese, red wine, and indulgent French food had taken its toll on my waistline (I peaked at 80kg and 36inch waist). Around that time the latest 'fad' was the Atkins diet. Robert Atkins was an American physician and cardiologist, born in 1930, who published his first book as early at 1972. It wasn't until the early years of the new millennium, however, that his ideas started to gain mainstream popularity. At one point nearly 10% of Americans admitted to being on some form of low-carb, Atkins style, diet. Krispy Kreme even blamed the diet for a fall in sales of their doughnuts.

The Atkins diet was originally considered unhealthy and demonised by the mainstream health authorities, mostly due to its high saturated fat content. If you recall, there has been a lot of misinformation around saturated fats – much of it originating directly or indirectly from Big Food who want to push their low-fat high-sugar agenda. There is now compelling evidence from respected studies that the right kinds of saturated fat are in fact harmless and even beneficial.

The Atkins diet has been studied thoroughly and shown to lead to more weight loss and greater improvements in blood sugar, 'good' HDL cholesterol, triglycerides, and other health markers than low-fat diets. Despite being high in fat, it does not raise 'bad' LDL cholesterol on average, though this does happen in a subset of individuals. The main reason why low-carb diets are so effective for weight loss is that a reduction in carbs and increased protein intake lead to reduced appetite, making you eat fewer calories without having to think about it.

My own personal experience of Atkins was very positive. I did not feel overly hungry, like you can with some diets, I could continue to eat lots of quality meat and fish and even drink a few glasses of red wine whilst still losing weight. Admittedly the diet is harder to follow for vegetarians but for many it proved to be a highly effective way of quickly shedding excess pounds. There was one group, however, who were not so keen on Atkins: Big Food.

An industry that is largely based around selling cheap, processed carbohydrates not surprisingly started briefing strongly against the Atkins diet. Some companies did initially try to exploit the trend by producing 'low-carb' versions of their brands. This approach was never going to be sustainable, so the focus quickly shifted to discrediting both Atkins and his theories. One conspiracy theory even put the blame for Atkins 'premature' death at the age of 72 on his low-carb diet. Robert Atkins actually died as a result of slipping on an icy pavement in New York and sustaining a fatal brain injury. The relentless PR attack from the food industry combined with Americans' well-ingrained habits and love of junk food meant that the Atkins diet eventually went the same way as other fad diets. I firmly believe that many of Atkins theories remain valid and that a fundamental switch away from carbs to healthy fats is a highly effective and healthy way to lose weight.

A few years later I started to take an interest in the lifestyle musings of Tim Ferriss, an American entrepreneur and author. In his bestselling, iconoclastic book 'The 4-hour Body' he covers a range of physiological topics from orgasms to muscle gain and most importantly weight loss. He skilfully explodes the myth that all calories are equal. They are not - 100 calories from beef is not the same as 100 calories from whisky (or bourbon as he prefers to call it). More pertinently the body responds differently to different food groups: the hormonal responses to carbohydrates, protein and fat are different. The slow-carb diet that Tim advocates is beautiful in its simplicity (and I can testify, along with many others, that it works). There are just 5 rules:

1. Avoid white carbohydrates (bread, rice, pasta, etc.)
2. Eat the same few meals over and over again
3. Don't drink calories
4. Don't eat fruit (except tomatoes and avocadoes)
5. Take one day off per week and eat whatever you want

I would advise you to buy the book to get the detail behind the above but the striking thing for me is the overlap with Atkins. Cutting out processed carbohydrates (rule 1) is the single best move you can make to lose weight and improve your diet and many of the foods he recommends are low GI. It also raises serious questions about PHE's 'Eatwell' guidance with its emphasis on 5 pieces of fruit and veg a day and support of starchy carbs (albeit wholegrain and high fibre). I believe PHE have got it wrong whereas Dr. Atkins and Ferriss are on the right track.

The other 'expert' who has greatly influenced my thinking is the author of 'The Fast Diet', Dr. Michael Mosley. This is an extract from the introduction to the revised edition of his seminal work:

'Over the last few decades, food fads have come and gone, but the standard medical advice on what constitutes a healthy lifestyle has stayed much the same: eat low-fat foods, exercise more... and never, ever skip meals. Over that same period levels of obesity have soared. Now many of those old certainties are being questioned.'

The basic premise of Dr. Mosley's '5:2' diet is to restrict calories (i.e. to fast) twice a week and on the remaining 5 days to eat normally. He recommends restricting calorie intake on fasting days to 600 for men and 500 for women. The good news is that by following the 5:2 regime you will experience benefits over and above mere weight loss. The long-term gains are potentially huge, cutting your risk of a range of diseases, including diabetes, heart disease and cancer. I have been experimenting with fasting, on and off, for the last few years. I follow 5:2 to lose weight (usually after Christmas!) and switch to 6:1 for weight maintenance. I have also experimented with a combination of Tim Ferris's slow-carb diet and 5:2 fasting with good results.

Whether you choose Atkins, slow-carb, 5:2 or a combination of all three, the common denominator is a significant reduction in carbohydrates and sugar, i.e. the very thing that the food industry has got you addicted to over many years. The good news is you can re-educate your palate over time to accept less sugar and processed carbs. A low-carb diet also doesn't need to be boring or bland. I consume the following foods on a regular (once a week or more) cycle:

- Free range eggs (for breakfast most days)
- Fillet steak (grass fed or organic)
- Free range or organic chicken breast
- Sea bass

143

- Peanut butter (no-added sugar, my preferred brand is Whole Earth Organic)
- Green & red lentils
- Olive oil, coconut oil (for cooking & salads)
- Nuts (Brazil, cashew, pecan, walnut)
- Sauerkraut (ideally organic fermented)
- Prawns
- Serrano or Parma ham
- Fresh tuna
- Unpasteurised cheese

Replacing refined carbs with high quality protein (lean meat, fish, or vegetables) is one of the keys to a healthy diet.

(NB. Both 'The Four Hour Body' and 'The Fast Diet' provide a range of recipes to suit all palates)

The other main overlap between the theories of Ferriss and Mosley is in their approach to exercise. Ferriss talks about Minimum Effective Dose (MED), while Mosley is an advocate of High Intensity Training (HIT). MED and HIT are essentially two sides of the same coin and both have the huge plus of making your exercise regime as effective and time efficient as possible. Combining a healthy diet with regular exercise will deliver the best overall results but remember 'you can't outrun a bad diet'. I put the emphasis at around 80:20 in favour of diet.

There are some sceptics who will read this chapter and question the science and data behind my assertions. The fact is that there are many thousands of people who have successfully followed the advice of Atkins, Ferriss and Mosley to achieve their weight goals (in Ferriss' case this also includes the small group of people looking to gain weight). In reality, many of the above theories will only be definitively proved correct in 10-20 years time, when currently on-going research projects are concluded. That is the nature of research into diet and nutrition – there are no quick answers. So, you have a choice. You can wait for that research to come out or you can go for immediate results with proven strategies. I think it is an easy call.

Conclusion

Here in the UK, we are extremely fortunate to live in a first world country with well-stocked, affordable supermarkets offering a wide variety of food products all year round. The food industry (comprising both manufacturers and retailers) is a major employer and its importance was brought into stark relief during the outbreak of the coronavirus when, after initial shortages caused by panic buying, the food supply chain stood resolutely up to the challenge of keeping the country fed. This is testament not only to robust systems and processes but also to the talented professional leaders within the industry (some of whom are my former colleagues).

So why do I consider these very same people to be, at least in part, responsible for the obesity crisis? The truth is that many of them become captured by the system in which they work. They grow to accept the corporate doctrine and prevailing attitudes within the food industry – the no bad foods, calories-in calories-out, balanced diet, healthy lifestyle doctrine. They start to believe the PR spin of their external affairs department. They successfully lobby against government intervention on the grounds of choice and personal freedom. I once asked a senior executive at British American Tobacco how he could sell a product that killed people. He replied, 'You sell Mars bars, they kill people too.' I laughed it off at the time, but I now realise he was right.

In this book I have focused on Britain's biggest food brands. Why? Because by definition they are what we buy and eat the most. There is a direct correlation between the biggest sellers and the biggest impact on the nation's health. What has become clear to me, however, is that we need to do what the food industry refuses to do and admit the real truth about how people are consuming their products. The marketers at Coca Cola know, but won't acknowledge, that for lunch you eat a bag of Walkers with your full-sugar Coke, plant-bread sandwich and a bar of Cadburys Dairy Milk. Heinz are indifferent to the fact that you put their ketchup on your McCain oven chips with Birds Eye fish fingers and will have a Mueller yoghurt for dessert and a Kit Kat before bed. Kellogg's are fully aware of the schoolboy who has a big bowl of Crunchy Nut Cornflakes for breakfast and swigs a Red Bull on his way to school with a Nestlé Yorkie so that he has had more than his safe level of sugar before he sits down for his first lesson. When challenged, all of these manufacturers will give essentially the same defence: 'our products are meant to be consumed as part of a balanced diet combined with a healthy lifestyle' is what they all say. It is a get out of jail card for all of the junk food producers complicit in the developing obesity scandal. There is safety in numbers – it is impossible to pin the blame on one manufacturer because the damage to our health comes from the cumulative effect of our consumption of a smorgasbord of junk food, not just one discrete product or brand. Everybody is responsible but no one is accountable.

The parallels with tobacco are irrefutable but there are also some significant differences. Cigarettes are essentially homogenous, highly addictive products that were proven to cause ill-health (i.e. lung disease). It still took years of medical research and expensive court cases to establish the facts and restrict the marketing of cigarettes through regulatory control (NB. They can still be legally purchased by anyone over 18). The challenge for governments seeking to tackle obesity is much harder. The food industry can and does hide behind its diversity and its popularity. Politicians won't win many votes by telling people to stop eating the food they like. Surely people should be allowed to make their own food choices in a liberal country like ours they argue? This explains why many public initiatives behind healthy eating are half-hearted and ineffective. It is also why PHE's dietary guidance (Eatwell) is so woefully inappropriate.

Meanwhile the strain on the NHS from obesity-related illnesses has surpassed that of smoking. Ironically, the majority of NHS workers are themselves overweight! [1] Yes, in theory we should be free to make our own choices. But what happens when many of us, encouraged by the food industry, continually make the wrong choices? You aren't allowed to drive your car at 100mph. So why should you be free to make yourself obese? The time has come for more paternalistic approaches with the nation's diet. The sugar tax on drinks is a start but we need more such measures, implemented quickly without any brakes applied by Big Food. This may happen eventually, but I wouldn't hold your breath. Governments tend to do what is popular not what's right. If I were advising government, I would give them the following 5-point plan:

1. Taxes on junk food

I know this is a blunt instrument, but it would work. Build on the learnings from the sugar tax on soft drinks and rollout to other categories starting with confectionery, crisps, and biscuits. I know such taxes are regressive but so are the duties on tobacco.

2. Educate children on food values

Make the studying of food, nutrition, and cookery compulsory in schools (minimum

GCSE level). It is far more relevant than algebra and will teach life skills and knowledge that are invaluable.

3. **Significantly restrict the availability of junk food.**

Ban junk from vending machines and remove from all government & council buildings like leisure centres and hospitals. Restrict sales in newsagents and other non-food outlets. Limit the amount of shelf space and ban promotions (e.g. BOGOFs) on junk food in supermarkets.

4. **Give the current regulatory bodies (ASA, FSA) more power to tackle the causes of obesity.**

There is currently too much consultation with the food industry, which succeeds in delaying and watering down government initiatives. The FSA should be able to mandate health warnings on junk food packaging, cf. the stark warnings on cigarette packs. The ASA should have the authority to ban junk food brands sponsoring sport and advertising at sports venues. More radically, the ASA should consider banning all junk food advertising (it is currently only banned for children). If it cannot decide what's junk, then it could start by reading this book.

5. **Incentivise everyone to stay within their healthy BMI range.**

Unlike the other measures above this is about carrot not stick. Give a specific 'NHS' tax allowance for those people who are within the healthy range. There would inevitably be issues around collecting and validating the data but with the technology available today it should be perfectly feasible. This is not about fat-shaming overweight people. If you are a healthy weight you are almost certainly going to be less of a drain on the NHS so why should you pay the same taxes as an obese person?

You might think that the above measures are too draconian and counter to the British tradition of liberal values and free choice. The fact is that people are increasingly choosing the SO-BAD approach. We need more radical solutions – more of the same tinkering won't work. Everyone wants to be free to choose until they become ill through obesity – then they want the state (i.e. the NHS) to save them. This cycle must be broken. Prevention has always been better than cure.

The good news is that if you follow the advice in this book you won't need to wait for the state's intervention. If there is one overriding message that you should heed, it is this:

Reduce the amount of processed food in your diet

A lot of processed food is junk, and all junk food is processed. I guarantee that by reducing the junk you will significantly improve your health, wellbeing, and your wallet. Start by making some easy changes, e.g. cutting out one or two of the junk categories from your weekly shop, then build up over time so that your shopping trolley eventually contains more non-processed food than processed. Within a matter of weeks, you will begin to notice a positive difference and your trips to the supermarket will help prolong your life instead of shortening it.

Happy Shopping!

RECOMMENDED READING

'Happy Food', Niklas Ekstedt & Henrik Ennart
'Swallow This', Joanna Blythman
'Salt, Sugar, Fat, How the Food Giants Hooked Us',
Michael Moss
'The Four Hour Body', Tim Ferris
'The Fast Diet', Dr. Michael Mosley & Mimi
Spencer

NOTES

Introduction

1. Statistics on Obesity, Physical Activity and Diet, England, 2019 (NHS Digital, 8 May 2019)

Chapter 1: The Crisis. Right here, right now

1. Obesity Indicators 2018, Scottish Government Statistics (30 October 2018)
2. Obesity Facts, Centers for Disease Control & Prevention (27 February 2020)
3. Why Is the Obesity Rate So Low in Japan and High in the U.S.? Some Possible Economic Explanations, Benjamin Senauer & Masahiko Gemma (2006)
4. World Health Organisation, Obesity Data & Statistics, (2020)

Chapter 2: Movers & Shakers in the UK Grocery industry

1. Food & Drink Industry Report 2020, Food & Drink Federation (2020)

2. www.tesco.com\about

Chapter 3: The Marketing of Food

1. Consumption of high-fructose corn syrup in beverages may play a role in the epidemic of obesity, The American Journal of Clinical Nutrition, (1 April 2004)
2. Does Sugar Addiction Really Cause Obesity? National Center for Biotechnology Information, Achim Peters, (13 January 2012)
3. Acrylamide levels in potato crisps in Europe from 2002 to 2016, Food Additives & Contaminants, S. Powers, D. Mottram, A. Curtis, N. Halford, (27 September 2017)

Chapter 4: The Killer Categories

1. Thermal Degradation of Vegetable Oils: Spectroscopic Measurement and Analysis, H. Vaskova & M. Buckova, Science Direct (2015)
2. Why nutritionists are crazy about nuts, Harvard Health Publishing (June 2017)
3. www.nhs.co.uk

Conclusion

1. Obesity prevalence among healthcare professionals in England: a cross-sectional study using the Health Survey for England, BMJ Open, R.G. Kyle (December 2017)

Printed in Great Britain
by Amazon